The Essential Skills for Setting Up a Counselling and Psychotherapy Practice

Many practitioners consider setting up in private practice at some point in their career, whether full-time or alongside other employment. *The Essential Skills for Setting up a Counselling and Psychotherapy Practice* provides comprehensive yet accessible coverage of all the major skills needed to succeed.

Based on the authors' extensive experience, this book provides a valuable insight into how to minimise the risks associated with working privately, offering practical advice on how to keep a balance between self-development, personal health and meeting the needs of clients, whilst maintaining high standards and making a reasonable living.

Acknowledging the fact that being a good therapist may not, in itself, be sufficient to be successful in self-employment, the authors discuss the need for sound business skills, professional development, self-knowledge and motivation. Divided into three parts, the book covers all the essential business, professional and personal skills and includes discussion of subjects such as **insurance, finance, legal issues, marketing, stress management, security** and **retirement planning**.

The focus on skills and how to acquire and develop them makes this book an invaluable reference for all mental health professionals who are considering setting up their own private practice.

Gladeana McMahon is Co-Director of the Centre for Stress Management and a psychotherapist in private practice.
Stephen Palmer is Director of the Centre for Stress Management and Honorary Professor of Psychology, City University, London.
Christine Wilding is a CBT psychotherapist in the private and corporate sectors.

The Essential Skills for Setting Up a Counselling and Psychotherapy Practice

Gladeana McMahon, Stephen Palmer
and Christine Wilding

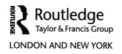

Routledge
Taylor & Francis Group

LONDON AND NEW YORK

First published 2005
by Routledge
27 Church Road, Hove, East Sussex BN3 2FA

Simultaneously published in the USA and Canada
by Routledge
270 Madison Ave, New York, NY 10016

Routledge is an imprint of the Taylor & Francis Group

Typeset in Times by Keystroke, Jacaranda Lodge, Wolverhampton
Printed and bound in Great Britain by MPG Books Ltd, Bodmin, Cornwall
Paperback cover design by Lisa Dynan

This publication has been produced with paper manufactured to strict
environmental standards and with pulp derived from sustainable forests.

British Library Cataloguing in Publication Data
A catalogue record for this book is available from the British Library

Library of Congress Cataloging in Publication Data
McMahon, Gladeana, 1954–
  The essential skills for setting up a counselling and psychotherapy
practice / Gladeana McMahon, Stephen Palmer, Christine Wilding.
     p. cm.
  Includes bibliographical references and index.
  ISBN 0-415-19775-9 – ISBN 0-415-19776-7 (pbk.) 1. Counseling.
2.Psychotherapy. I. Palmer, Stephen, 1955- II. Wilding, Christine.
III.Title.

  BF637.C6M3797 2005
  616.89'0068–dc22   2004024324

ISBN 0–415–19775–9 hbk
ISBN 0–415–19776–7 pbk

Contents

Preface

An acquaintance of one of the authors threw over a secure well-paid professional job to run a flower shop – something she had always dreamed of doing.

There was very little she didn't know about flowers. She had taken extensive lessons from acknowledged experts in flower arranging. She was well versed in the purchase, care and culture of flowers. Yet, within eighteen months, deep in debt and her dreams shattered, she was obliged to sell up and return to the profession she had left.

Her case is not unique. Each year, thousands of businesses, large and small, cease trading.

Many therapists engaged in or contemplating private practice do not appreciate that being a good therapist may not, in itself, be sufficient to make a successful career in self-employment. The development of business skills, continued professional development, self-knowledge and motivation are also key factors in success.

More therapists are trained each year than there are counselling jobs to take them. While a number of people want to use their counselling training to enhance another job such as social work or teaching, there are still a significant number who are surprised and disappointed to find that it is hard to make the career change they had hoped for. For some, the idea of self-employment is often turned to as the only way of being able to earn an income doing a job they have been trained to do, rather than because it is a positive career progression or choice. Even therapists who have many years' experience and excellent qualifications and a proven track record can find making a living from private practice difficult. You only need to open any local telephone directory to see that there are many therapists of all orientations and titles (psychologists, counsellors, psychotherapists, hypnotherapists) advertising their services either as individuals or as part of a fee-paying organisation.

A student contacted one of the authors for careers advice during the last six months of his two-year diploma course. He had used the redundancy money from his job as a computer programmer in the private sector to finance the course. He had used his time and money to gain as much experience as he could in a variety of voluntary sector placements during his course and had accrued a large number of counselling hours in a range of settings.

As the second year of his course progressed he turned his attention towards the matter of preparing himself for employment. However, he discovered that there were very few paid jobs available and those that were advertised asked for accredited or registered therapists. He became increasingly despondent as the prospect that he might have to take a non-counselling job to pay his bills became a necessity. Not surprisingly he turned his thoughts towards the idea of becoming self-employed. He believed that this option would provide the opportunity of using his skills while making the income he needed to survive. Following a series of meetings the student realised that he did not really want to become self-employed, as he did not feel he was ready for all that such a career option entailed. Instead he chose to take a part-time job that would allow him to earn enough money to get by while he invested in his counselling future by continuing to work in a voluntary capacity to increase his experience and work towards becoming accredited. Six months later one of the voluntary agencies he had been working for was able to attract enough funding to take on another full-time counsellor/administrator, and much to his relief he got the job.

It is the purpose of this book to provide an understanding of what is needed to be successful in private practice and to give practical guidance in the development of those skills essential for success.

Introduction

WHO IS THE BOOK FOR?

In 1994 Gladeana McMahon wrote a teach-yourself manual, *Setting Up Your Own Private Practice in Counselling and Psychotherapy*. The manual was seminal and remains, to the best of our knowledge, the only UK publication of its type and format dealing with private practice. It has been and still is extensively used in workshops and training courses. A decade later this book aims to bring together the current thinking, expertise and skills to become a successful self-employed professional.

Although counselling and psychotherapy remain the professional focus of the book, it may also be of use to psychologists, hypnotherapists, alternative health practitioners, and most therapists already in private practice. Given the possibility of a wide range of readers we will use the word therapist to denote the practitioner. The business sections of the book in particular are also relevant for many self-employed people in terms of the marketing, financial and administrative skills required.

EMPHASIS ON SKILLS AND PRACTICE

This book focuses on *skills* and *how to acquire them* through knowledge, experience and practice. Theoretical argument and discussion are kept to a minimum and this is reflected in the use of fewer references than one would normally expect. This demonstrates the authors' desire to make this a practical rather than an academic book. Those references that are included are generally restricted to those publications where practical guidance and advice can be found. There is a recommended reading section at the end of the book for those who wish to pursue individual aspects in greater depth.

CONFLICTS INVOLVED IN PRIVATE PRACTICE

As in many professions, there are always conflicts between personal needs, professional ethics and integrity, political or religious beliefs and the achievement of acceptable standards of living for the practitioner.

Of course, even paid employment frequently involves conflict. Many people suffer stress, working long hours in jobs where the pressures are difficult to cope with, where they have little control over day-to-day events, in unsatisfactory relationships with bosses or colleagues or where there is little sense of achievement. Families, a social life and personal health can be ignored until it is too late.

In private practice some of these pressures are relieved, but replaced by others. Your time may be your own but you must use it to create and meet a demand for your services. You do not have an employer who will provide paid work, paid holidays, paid sick or maternity leave, working premises, equipment, materials, pension schemes, training, etc. You may work largely in isolation without the support of colleagues. Worries about redundancy are replaced by concerns over not generating sufficient income to survive and meet your outgoings. Standards of practice and ethics are for you to decide. You may feel uneasy or guilty about charging clients who can ill afford your fees, or actually turning away someone because they cannot pay at all.

You alone have to take responsibility for building and sustaining a credible and acceptable professional reputation. You can run risks of personal safety in dealing with disturbed clients. Perhaps you are hopeless with paperwork, record-keeping and accounts. How do you keep a balance between self-development, personal health, and meeting the needs of clients, while maintaining high standards and making a reasonable living? We shall address all of these issues.

THE NEED FOR PREPARATION TO AVOID DISAPPOINTMENT AND BANKRUPTCY

In the United States there is not the same stigma or penalty attached to bankruptcy (i.e. being unable to pay your debts), and many previously bankrupted Americans have gone on to be successful. Their business culture is more geared to risk-taking than ours is and it can be easier to bounce back, having learned the valuable lessons associated with failure. However, while it is undoubtedly true that some of the most useful lessons are learnt from taking risks and making mistakes, we would not recommend bankruptcy as a serious option. It has been said that risks can be classified in three ways:

- *Risks you can afford to take.* For example, you have a client who has failed to respond to a particular approach. You consider using an alternative approach that also has a risk of failure. None the less, you are justified in trying it.
- *Risks you cannot afford to take.* For example, you are female and are offered a client with a history of serious assault against women. You work on your

own and you decide not to accept the referral and instead recommend an alternative agency.

- *Risks you cannot afford not to take*. For example, you have a significant number of clients on low fees. In an attempt to meet your financial outgoings you find yourself seeing more clients than you can comfortably manage and have little time for anything else. You know you should reduce the number of clients and raise your fees but fear a drop in business. You reduce client numbers and raise fees.

Much of this book is concerned with turning unmanaged risks into managed risks, reducing uncertainty and enabling private practice therapists to take more control of their chosen profession. Risks are unavoidable but, unless you are an inveterate gambler willing to stake everything on the turn of a card, you are likely to be happier and more confident knowing that you are following sound business, professional and ethical principles.

Good preparation benefits a whole range of activities – whether it is sitting for an exam, acting in a play, applying for a job, running in a race or going on holiday. Preparation reduces unnecessary risks. Spending time now can save time later and prevent panic. Good preparation does not eliminate the unexpected but does create more time for dealing with it when it happens.

If you are thinking of setting up your own private practice, good preparation will undoubtedly improve your chances of success. As to what you need to prepare, this is covered in the sections that follow.

PART ONE

The business skills

WHAT MAKES SOME BUSINESSES SUCCESSFUL AND OTHERS FAIL?

This is a fundamental question on which many books have been written and will continue to be written. Most people will be aware of the closure of coalmines, steelworks or shipyards and have noticed shops boarded up in depressed areas. What is not so visible is the failure of many small businesses run from private homes or small premises. It is not that such businesses necessarily go bankrupt, rather that the owners give up as they see the inevitability of bankruptcy, in an attempt to cut their losses.

Yet in many cases such disappointments are avoidable. The first useful business skill to be acquired lies in your ability to appreciate what makes the difference between success and failure, and in applying this knowledge to your own private practice.

First, it is worth looking at some of the reasons why a private practice may fail.

Why practices fail

The original idea was not thought through

When his partner left him, Alan remained in a nicely furnished two-bedroom flat on the eighth floor of a tower block. An accredited therapist, he decided to convert the second bedroom into a consulting room and office and start his own private practice. Three months later he gave up paid employment and started advertising for clients.

The initial response was good and his appointment book started filling up. However, he was surprised at the number of potential clients who never turned up for the first meeting and also at how very few clients, particularly women, persisted beyond the first one or two sessions.

He discussed his cases and his concerns with his supervisor. He shared his thoughts with a colleague and it was his colleague who pointed out the possibility that the unattractive environment where Alan lived could be part of the problem. The lift was often out of order, there was graffiti and although there was never any real trouble there were some dubious characters hanging around. Alan had failed to see his environment through the eyes of his potential clients and realised he could not run a successful practice from his present home.

When Alan rented a room at a local complementary health centre he found his clients turned up and stayed the course.

Insufficient income

Lucy was a lone parent who ran a busy private practice while her daughter was at school. Typically, she was able to see five clients a day, five days a week, for forty weeks in the year. Most of her clients could afford no more than between £10 and £15 per session. After subtracting the costs of running her business, Lucy realised that she would be just as well off drawing unemployment and other related benefits. She gave up private practice and joined a voluntary organisation as a paid therapist.

Insufficient working capital

Hearing of the experiences of Alan and Lucy, Katherine was determined to learn from their experiences to make a success of private practice. She found premises in a very pleasant location at a rent of £400 per month and signed a twelve-month tenancy agreement. She saw her bank manager and managed to get an unsecured loan of £4,000 repayable over two years; £3,000 of the loan went on the deposit on the premises, a computer, furniture and furnishings and general office items, leaving £1,000 'to be on the safe side'. She decided she would charge clients £25 per session.

Katherine had moved back home to live with her parents when her relationship broke down and she reckoned she could manage on living expenses of £500 a month. Her parents were happy to support her in her business venture as they could see the long-term advantages for their daughter. What could go wrong?

Clients started arriving, paid their fees and remained for repeat sessions. Katherine felt encouraged. However, although client numbers were steadily increasing they were not doing so as quickly as Katherine had imagined they would. She was surprised at how quickly the spare £1,000 from her bank loan disappeared, even though she had been very strict with her own personal expenditure.

After three months Katherine had run out of cash and was concerned with regard to her tenancy agreement. She reviewed her income and expenditure. Her records showed:

Income (3 months)		Expenditure (3 months)	
		Deposit on premises	£400
Month 1 – 16 sessions	£400	Rent	£1,200
Month 2 – 24 sessions	£600	Loan repayments	£580
Month 3 – 40 sessions	£1,000	Telephone bills	£200
		Living expenses	
		(Drawings)	£1,500
Sub-total	£2,000	Sub-total	£3,880
Deficit financed by:			
Remaining bank loan	£1,000		
Personal savings	£880		
Total	£3,880	Total	£3,880

Faced with a drop in income over the Christmas period, the cancellation of a skiing holiday in January, the exhaustion of her own remaining personal savings and the probable sale of her car, Katherine approached her landlord, who agreed to cancel her lease in return for retaining the initial deposit. The bank loan repayments were rescheduled over a longer time period and Katherine arranged for colleagues to take over her clients.

Insufficient financial control

Nicole was a very popular therapist and she had no problem keeping her clients even though her fees were high, but she was not very good at bookkeeping and at year-end there was a mad panic to sort out her accounts. Although she had worked on a range of personal issues in her own therapy, her impoverished childhood still showed itself in her wallet full of credit cards being used to the limit.

Needless to say, matters took a turn for the worse when demands for payment were not met. Fortunately, she acquired a business partner who took control of the financial side of the business.

Insufficient skills

Arthur was in his early fifties and, although he had no formal training in counselling, he helped out in his spare time at his local church and for various charities. People found him an empathic and helpful person and he was seen as an asset to the organisations he worked for. His clerical job in local government gave him no satisfaction and when he was made redundant he decided to convert his deceased mother's bedroom into a consulting room and advertise his services as a therapist.

Arthur had no idea of what he should be charging or how to deal with the majority of clients who came his way. The realities of working with a range of clients challenged his abilities and this saddened him because he had thought he would be able to offer a good service to his clients. He soon came to realise that he was out of his depth and, feeling shaken and demoralised, he gave up his private work.

Lack of motivation and energy

Patrick was a laid-back therapist always putting off 'till tomorrow what he should do today'. Early-morning clients would sometimes surprise him before he had dressed or washed. His consulting room was a mess for which he was always apologising. Client files were left lying around and one client took great exception to this and complained to Patrick's professional association about his behaviour. The resulting investigation was more than he could handle; he gave up counselling and drifted into a series of part-time jobs.

Hard-working and conscientious to the point of breakdown

Petra took on every client who came her way, most with deep-seated problems. She found it hard not to feel personally responsible and was conscientious in the extreme. Her clients could ring her at any time and did, frequently late at night. Although she was working with her supervisor on the issue of therapeutic boundaries, she was finding this a difficult issue to manage. Over a five-year period, due to circumstances outside her control, she received supervision from four different supervisors and the issue of therapeutic boundaries never got resolved.

In the end, Petra suffered from burnout and her income dried up as she felt unable to cope with client work. She took a routine nine-to-five job where she could switch off when her work was over and devote more time to her own needs.

Family pressures

Jane decided to run her own practice when both her children were at primary school. She was well organised and the extra money helped to pay for holidays, home improvements and treats for the children. Although reluctant at first, her husband was happy that she was finding fulfilment in her counselling work, and it took the pressure off him to be the sole provider. Jane's mother lived nearby and helped out with the children during the holidays.

This arrangement worked well until Jane's mother suffered a stroke and wasn't able to help out. The children wanted their friends to visit and it was difficult to contain the noise in a small house. The hours Jane was able to devote to clients in a peaceful atmosphere reduced to the point where it was hardly worth the effort. It became very difficult to manage family and client needs at the same time. In the end Jane gave up her private practice but resolved to return to it when the children had effectively left home.

The wrong location

Jack was a keen sailor with his own boat. He devoted weekends, holidays and most of his spare money to sailing. When the opportunity came to move to a seaside resort with a marina, Jack jumped at the chance.

Up to that time Jack had worked as a self-employed therapist in a large city, where the problem was how to fit in the large numbers of clients who presented themselves. Starting again in the more relaxed environment of a seaside town with a large population of older retired people, Jack was surprised at the small number of clients he was able to attract.

In a bid to drum up more business, he cut his fees substantially, but with little effect. There just didn't seem to be the same demand for fee-paying counselling services. Fortunately, his sea-going and boat-repair skills were in great demand and sufficient to provide a modest living.

Bad luck

Elspeth was set for a promising career in private practice counselling. Talented and hard-working, she had everything going for her.

One summer's evening, driving home, she collided with a stolen car driven through red lights by two teenagers. Apart from the severe physical injuries that stopped her working for six months, she also suffered from post-traumatic stress disorder, which completely undermined her self-confidence, and she experienced frequent panic attacks together with a range of other symptoms that prevented her from doing counselling work for a long time afterwards.

Conclusion

The above vignettes illustrate some of the reasons why a private practice may fail. Although, clearly, they are not comprehensive, it can be seen that a number of factors are involved in the provision of a successful practice. These include personal factors, such as the motivation and skills of the therapist, financial factors, such as the generation of sufficient income and the control of expenses, and environmental factors such as location and ambience.

All these factors and more will be covered in this section. First, let's look at the personal characteristics of a successful business person and see what relevance these might have for a therapist running a private practice.

The personal characteristics of a successful business person

Having your own business is one thing. Running it successfully is another. What personal factors distinguish the successful from the less successful (Caird, 1993; Gordon, 1984)?

Drive

Personal motivation and drive are essential qualities: you must want to succeed and be prepared to put the work into your practice. People with drive and motivation are likely to view obstacles and failures as challenges rather than as distressing setbacks. You will need to believe in yourself and in your ability to provide services that clients will perceive as good value for money.

Logical and creative thinking

Many of you will have seen television programmes about companies (usually, but not always, small ones) in difficulties, including the 'trouble-shooter' series with John Harvey-Jones. In many such cases, the owners and managers are hard-working and forever optimistic but that is not enough to stop them getting into difficulties.

Successful business people have the ability to look objectively and logically at their business, to be aware of the key priorities, to balance immediate needs and longer-term goals, to know when detail can be critical or just a distraction, to distinguish between the essential and the desirable.

Creativity is important in generating alternatives, some of which may be better options than the current policy or practice. The combination of logical analysis and creative thinking is even more powerful, as many therapists will be aware through their analysis of client problems and the generation of alternative thinking or behaviours.

Sometimes, apparently good ideas need testing in practice. Good businesses are always testing new markets or new products, preferably before their competitors. Many of these come to nothing and you have probably noticed products that appear briefly on the supermarket shelves only to disappear again. None the less, some will be very successful. If nothing is tried, nothing is gained. In therapy, decisions need to be taken about the type of clientele one is aiming at, the choice of therapeutic approach, the style of communication with potential clients and many other factors. Some experimentation may be required before the best options are reached. The determination of the cost effectiveness of different forms of advertising is an obvious example.

Acceptable risk-taking

Life is full of risks, and insurance companies do very nicely out of our fear of something happening to our families, our possessions or us.

Sometimes, the greatest risk is to do nothing and, sometimes, the greater risk is to tinker with a perfectly good business. Newly appointed chief executives can be prone to this when they perceive a need to establish their own authority by restructuring, out-sourcing, or by adopting the most recent 'flavour of the month' management techniques.

The technique known as 'risk assessment', though, probably has some validity.

Good businesses can become outdated or undermined by competitors. Knowledge advances inexorably and those that acquire and, more importantly, are able to apply up-to-date knowledge can secure a premium for their services.

The capacity for taking risks is very much an individual characteristic. However, the end result is invariably improved by careful analysis and good judgement. Fallback positions if things go wrong should be determined in advance to prevent subsequent panic or over-hasty actions under pressure. It is a mark of a successful person to know when to cut losses and get out rather than persist with a lost cause. The maxim, 'when you have dug yourself into a hole, stop digging', is sensible advice. Even more sensible is to remember the ladder!

Running a therapy business should not be a gamble; neither should it be allowed to stagnate for a lack of sensible decisions.

Sometimes success breeds smugness and complacency. This can be very dangerous, as a number of leading British retailers have found out to their cost. It takes a long time to build a reputation for good-value products or services but only a short time to lose it.

The successful business person realises that continued success depends on continued objective appraisal of the business and current market forces. Success provides the opportunity, in terms of time and resources, to plan and implement improvements for still further success.

Business knowledge and skills

The previous section 'why businesses fail' provided a number of examples of people who may have been good therapists but because they lacked business knowledge and skills they failed in running a successful private practice.

Planning, organising and attention to detail

The advantage of having a plan is that it provides a means of measuring how good you are at forecasting and planning and, since plans invariably fail, in one respect or another, the reasons for failure are usually fairly clear. Lessons can be learned, adjustments can be made and, hopefully, techniques and decisions improved.

Imagine trying to sail around the world without a plan covering routes, times, supplies, communications, emergency procedures, training, etc. It is not unknown for people to try it but they invariably finish in disaster.

Military commanders provide numerous historic examples of good planning, organisation and attention to detail or, perhaps more commonly, the failure to plan or to appreciate when a plan is not working.

Although running a private practice does not involve the same life-or-death struggle as warfare, the same principles of planning, organising and attention to detail still apply. Opportunities need to be taken. The best use must be made of the resources available to you. Reserves, in the form of savings, overdraft facilities, and time (in the form of extra hours working), may sometimes need to be drawn upon.

Victories or successes need to be consolidated and built upon ready for the next campaign or business venture.

Reflection issues
- Measure your personal qualities against those of a successful business person. Which ones do you feel you have and which ones might you need to develop?
- Think about the reasons why practices might fail and think about whether you believe any of these factors apply to you.
- Consider therapists you personally know who are in private practice. What can you learn from them?

STARTING YOUR BUSINESS

Who can help?

Even if you are totally confident of making a success of private practice (perhaps even more so if you are already operating such a practice), it is wise to get as much informed advice and help as possible before you start. Where can you get such advice?

Other therapists and related professionals

If you have friends or colleagues in the same business and you are not setting up in direct competition with them, then their own experiences can be of assistance. They will know, for example, what fee levels are acceptable, what sort of clients they have and how far clients are prepared to travel. You can get ideas on how to attract clients. Perhaps you may even persuade them to refer surplus clients to you on the basis that one day you may be in a position to return the favour. In any event, it is helpful to belong to a professional support group since you may well be working in isolation for most of the time.

Friends and family

Friends and family may not be in a position to offer professional advice and, even if they were, you might not be prepared to take it. Clearly, if you have a partner or children or both, their needs must be taken into account. The personal, and perhaps financial, support, though, from a partner or close family can make a big difference to your venture and provide a useful base on which to build.

Banks

Banks are in the business of lending money for a profit. The bank manager or branch business adviser should therefore be able to appraise and assess business proposals objectively. A local bank is likely to have many small businesses as clients, possibly even therapists in private practice, and may well have a view as to the viability of your proposals should you need a loan or overdraft. If you do decide you need to borrow money to finance your business in the early stages, then try to obtain an overdraft facility rather than a loan or an unauthorised overdraft that will cost more, and earmark the money for specific business purposes.

Obtain alternative quotes and conditions – your own bank may not be the most competitive – and draw up a business plan in support of your proposal (more on this later).

Banks have come in for much criticism recently – overcharging, incompetence, bankrupting small businesses unnecessarily and being indifferent and unresponsive to complaints, to mention but a few. Like politicians, they tend to respect only those who wield similar levels of power. It has been said that if you owe a bank £1,000 it can make your life a misery but if you owe it £10 million you will receive courteous attention.

However, the high street banks do have a range of services available to help small business: for example, free financial computer software and leaflets, booklets and books on a range of issues relating to self-employment, as well as specialist staff able to help you design your business.

Accountants

Sooner or later you are likely to need an accountant, if only to audit your accounts. As a prospective client, an initial meeting (preferably with someone personally recommended) is likely to cost you very little or nothing at all. However, he/she can usually provide helpful advice on setting up your own business, for example:

- The different headings under which to record your expenditure.
- What expenditures are allowable for tax purposes and whether they are fully claimable in the current year or written down over a number of years.
- The financial records you need to keep.
- The use of bank or building society accounts for income, expenditure and making provision for tax.
- The pros and cons of using an online bank account.

Although most of these subjects are covered later, tax regulations can and do change and accountants are obliged to keep up to date. In addition to preparing your accounts, and with the advent of self-assessment in relation to taxation, an accountant can also complete the relevant documentation from the Inland Revenue on your behalf from the information you provide.

It is possible to do without the services of an accountant if your income is below £15,000 a year. If this is the case then you can prepare your own accounts and send these in to the Inland Revenue. This will save you money. However, you will not get the benefit of the up-to-date knowledge of tax breaks that an accountant will have.

Government-funded initiatives

Depending on the age of the applicant and the location of the business there are schemes (such as the Prince's Youth Business Trust for the under-thirties) and local funds available for business start-up.

At the local level, various initiatives exist to promote small business start-up and entrepreneurship in general. In some cities, specialised agencies have been set up to attract investment resources (grants, bank loans, etc.), which are used to support all small enterprises. These agencies are comparable to investment trusts. Some local authorities provide special refurbishment grants for small enterprises to upgrade their premises.

Business Link is a national business advice service that provides information on all business needs and access to a wide network of business support organisations.

Enterprise agencies exist to encourage new business and details can be obtained from your local reference library. Successive governments have often been criticised for making life difficult for small businesses, and the recent bringing forward of tax payments supports this view, in spite of the hot-air rhetoric to the contrary. However, enterprise agencies funded by both public and private sources can be helpful and frequently provide a free advice service. If you have been unemployed for three months but have some start-up capital, you may be eligible for an 'Enterprise Allowance', which lasts for one year and consists of weekly payments.

You can get further details on these and other such services by contacting your local authority, job centre or the Department of Trade and Industry.

Educational institutes, local councils, libraries, etc.

If you are a bit weak on the business side of running your own practice, then you may find some useful courses run by your local authority's further education institutes, such as bookkeeping and accounting, marketing, communications and publicity. Day or evening classes are frequently available and details can be obtained from your town hall or local library.

Some local authorities have an economic development department or, at least, officers who are concerned with reducing unemployment levels in the borough, who tend to work in association with agencies and employers. Government grants are often given to development agencies, particularly to regenerate previously deprived areas. Some local authorities own business premises that are available for rent, usually for less than a private sector letting.

As a private practitioner your business will depend on being able to attract significant numbers of clients able to pay your fees. While it is not too difficult to assess the general level of wealth in your catchment area from the proportion of good-quality privately owned houses, shops, cars, etc., the census statistics held by local planning departments (available for a fee) provide a breakdown of the various socio-economic groups. The reality of private practice is that your clients have to be able to afford your fees if you are to make an income.

Reflection issues
- What type of help might you need?
- Where will you find this help?
- What can you learn from other therapists?

A Business Plan

Introduction

Most successful businesses utilise a business plan as a means of setting objectives for the organisation and subsequently as a yardstick against which to measure performance and forecasting ability. It is from these starting points that the organisation's 'budgets' are derived – essentially, sales income, cost of sales, overheads and profit – and woe betide the sales and marketing managers who get their forecasts wrong! Central and local governments go through similar processes at least once a year, sometimes with intermediate reviews and adjustments.

As an individual running your own business, all this might seem like using the proverbial sledgehammer to crack a nut – after all, is not your main concern just to make enough money to live on, pay the mortgage, perhaps run a car and have a few holidays? Unfortunately, life is rarely that simple. You may have family commitments – to raise a child to adulthood (or beyond) can cost in the region of £50,000–£100,000. You may wish to retire at 60, 55 or even 50, and so may need to make large pension contributions to avoid relative poverty later on. Illness can strike at any time and deprive you of income. Then there is your professional development to consider – books, journals, courses, conferences, membership of professional bodies and so on. Such considerations should not be ignored. In a sense we are talking about your personal survival.

It can be difficult to separate your own personal requirements from those of your business – after all you are the business. Your own personal resources, skills and abilities make the business what it is. Your time is precious and should be utilised to achieve a balance between short-term, long-term and personal needs.

In planning your business it is helpful to have longer-term goals in mind. Do you want to work flat out for twenty years and then retire or do something different? Or would you prefer a less pressured existence with, perhaps, greater variety in the type of work you do? Do you have such a choice? What personal constraints do you operate under? Will they always be there?

You and your business are unique. Although there may appear to be a certain common daily routine – seeing and helping clients and dealing with your administration and finances – nothing stays the same for very long. Professionally, you will change as your experience grows. Clients' perceived problems and expectations will change as new or modified therapies are developed. Traditional therapist/client contact is already changing to include telephone counselling and the use of e-mail and the Internet. Short-term, action-orientated counselling is growing, with greater use of cognitive-behavioural techniques.

Enormous advances in the power of, and the variety of tasks undertaken with, electronic systems and equipment have already made and will continue to make an impact both on the potential efficiency of your business and on the sources, size and type of demand for your services.

Of course, it is not easy to project forward such trends to create a realistic scenario in which you may have to operate in, say, five or ten years' time, and, however hard you try, you won't get it exactly right. None the less, you should be aware of such developments and take account of them or make provision for them.

You may or may not remember that not so long ago many general practitioners operated as individuals without an appointment system, which was an inefficient use of their time as well as that of their patients. Now it seems almost inconceivable that anyone would operate in this way but at the time it seemed quite revolutionary for doctors to get together in a group practice to cover for each other and be able to employ professional administrative support staff to maximise doctor/patient contact time. However, some general practitioners are now reverting to the earlier system.

First steps in defining your business

In this and the following sections, the processes involved in business planning will be described (Barrow, 2001). It should perhaps be emphasised that there is no single 'golden road' to follow since all business plans should be geared to the circumstances, environment and resources prevailing for each business and to the nature and size of the potential market for its services. None the less, there are common threads in the creation of any business plan.

Step One – What business are you in?

A former management consultant said that his supervisor, in writing to a new client, would start a letter along the lines of 'Dear Mr Mackay, you are in the (fish curing) business. . . .' This sometimes produced a puzzled response from his clients, but he was unrepentant, claiming that many people did not know what business they were in. If you are a follower of the stock market you may remember that large conglomerates – companies comprising many divergent businesses – were all the rage in the 1980s – Hanson, BTR, Grand Metropolitan and BATS, for example. Now, these companies have either sold off non-core activities or been taken over or merged. Vertical integration, i.e. control of production, distribution and sometimes retailing, has also tended to give way to horizontal integration, i.e. taking over of direct competitors, whether in production, distribution or the supply of goods and services to end-users. The take-overs or mergers of banks, building societies, insurance companies, brewers, car manufacturers and communications companies have been particularly noticeable.

'What has all this got to do with me?' you may ask.

The answer lies in two parts.

First, both you and the chief executive of a multi-national company are constrained by time. In the course of a week you can give only limited consideration to a limited number of issues. If the issues are unrelated and call for different knowledge bases and skills, then you will struggle to succeed. Second, it is much easier to build on existing strengths in knowledge and skills than to acquire new knowledge and skills. GPs can cover for each other and so can airline pilots but to mix them up could be catastrophic.

The same arguments may be applied to therapy. Few therapists, if any, could deal successfully with children, severe mental health cases and psychotic clients unless specifically trained. This is not to say that it isn't possible to gain a good general appreciation of how to manage a wide spectrum of clients in therapy. It is, however, important that a therapist should, to paraphrase Clint Eastwood in the film *Dirty Harry*, 'know her/his own limitations'.

Of course, further specialised training and practical experience will expand skills and expertise, but a realistic assessment of one's own capabilities is essential.

How far you go down the road of defining your business is a matter of personal choice. Many examples are given in the *Counselling and Psychotherapy Resources Directory*, published by the British Association for Counselling and Psychotherapy, where a paragraph on each therapist normally contains the following information.

Registration:	professional organisations, if any, with which the therapist is registered
Code of ethics:	which organisations' codes of ethics are subscribed to
Qualifications & training:	self-explanatory, can also include accreditation
Personal therapy:	whether undertaken or not by the therapist
Supervision:	ongoing supervision arrangements
Service/ specialisation:	most therapists list general counselling and psychotherapy as a start and then list their own personal specialisms such

	as phobias, eating disorders, stress, relationships, work-related, depression, abuse, bereavement, etc.
Works with:	normally answered as: individuals, couples, families and/or groups
Clientele includes:	sometimes answered as 'anyone', but can include people in particular professions, children, young people, suicides, religious groups, sexual or ethnic minorities, people with disabilities, etc.
Theoretical orientation:	hundreds of listed approaches, the most common being psychodynamic, humanistic/person-centred, Rogerian/integrative, transpersonal and cognitive-behavioural
	Other languages: languages other than English offered by the therapist
Fees:	in the range of £10–80 per hour, typically £30–60 (in 2004)

All of the above helps to define the business you are in. Apart from direct therapy with clients, there may also be therapy-related activities that build on your existing skills as a therapist, such as giving talks, teaching, writing articles, chapters or books, media work and supervising other therapists.

You can, if you wish, attempt to summarise the above into a mission statement (though this term is no longer fashionable) such as:

> *To create and sustain a successful business through the provision of fully competent professional counselling and counselling-related services governed by the ethical requirements of the British Association for Counselling and Psychotherapy*

Step Two – Defining your resources

A successful business is one that manages to optimise the use of its own resources to match the needs of its customers, and so it is worthwhile to list what these resources actually are. They may be personal (knowledge, skills, personal stamina) or environmental (geographical location, easy access for clients, lack of competition, pleasant environment and facilities, etc.). None of these factors is usually represented on a balance sheet in monetary terms, though attempts are made from time to time in terms of goodwill (when a company is taken over at a higher value than its net assets) and the value of well-known brands.

Resources

A curriculum vitae (CV) is a useful starting point from which to extract information. The jobs you have held, qualifications attained, courses attended and your practical experience, all with the relevant dates, comprise the main elements. If you don't have a curriculum vitae then produce one and update it periodically. There are a number of excellent books that will help you do this, including *Creating a Successful CV* by Simon Howard. You never know when it will be needed at short notice, particularly if you want to do work for organisations. Don't forget to include any registrations or accreditations. If you have written any articles or contributed to any publications, list them.

The purpose of a CV or its equivalent, your Business Plan, is to sell yourself as a credible supplier of those services you are offering, and so it is worth the effort to make it presentable and up to date.

The services you are offering come next. These should be described in easy-to-understand, non-technical terms. The non-professional is unlikely to understand terms such as NLP, Gestalt or Winnicottian therapy. Even psychodynamic, person-centred or integrative therapy may cause problems. However, short-term or long-term counselling for adults with relationship problems should be readily understood.

Since most counselling involves travel by the client to see you, the location of your practice in terms of convenient access and a pleasant and safe environment for potential clients is a resource to be listed. Of course, with cheap access to the Internet and the use of online cameras, the day may come when location ceases to have such relevance, but not yet.

Step Three – Define the potential demand for your services

Is there likely to be sufficient demand for your services? This is *the* fundamental question. To answer it involves a number of stages.

Stage 1

Bearing in mind realistic travelling distances or times, how big is your potential market, i.e. how many people in your catchment area are in a position to use your services?

As far as we know, no one has as yet done the necessary market research to determine how many people in, say, the United Kingdom use therapy services in the course of a year and, of these, what share is served by private practitioners.

However, it is possible to do some very crude calculations based on rough statistics that are available. In 1999 there were about 5,000 therapists advertising their services in the *Counselling and Psychotherapy Resources Directory* or the National Register of Psychotherapists (after subtracting duplication and organisations) to a United Kingdom population of, say, 58 million, which means, on average, some 11,600 people per listed therapist. However, this average hides the geographical variation that exists, ranging from roughly 1 for 2,000 people in north-west London to 1 for 60,000 people in Scotland and Northern Ireland.

For private practices, there appears to be, not surprisingly, a very high correlation between the numbers of people with the ability to pay and the numbers of listed private practitioners. It is possible to attempt to be a little more precise. For example, the majority of clients are likely to be drawn from the AB socio-economic group (managers, administrative and professional), comprising perhaps 20 per cent of the population and, of these, most clients will be in the 20–60 age group, comprising perhaps 60 per cent of the population. Thus one could say there is a 'target' group of around 12 per cent of the general population. For this 'target' group, there is one therapist for about 1,400 people.

Of course, all the above is very approximate. There will be some clients from other socio-economic groups such as C1 (skilled workers); and not all practitioners will take on similar numbers of clients. Even within the AB group there will be some professions that use therapists more than others. One could also use a more typical age range of 25–50 years, and so on.

Stage 2

Until more research is done, there is little option but to do a calculation of the following type:

- Define your catchment area in terms of distance/time taken realistically for a client prepared to use your services. This could be 2–5 miles in a densely populated area with traffic problems or 10–30 miles in a rural district with clear roads, or, in time terms, up to one hour.
- Obtain the population figures for your catchment area. Local authority planning departments keep census figures. AA and Michelin guides also contain town populations.
- Try to find out the proportion of the catchment area population that is in the AB group. If this is not possible, compare the general wealth of the catchment area with other areas in terms of quality owner-occupied housing, new expensive cars, luxury shopping, etc. and adjust the AB figure of 20 per cent upwards or downwards accordingly.
- Multiply the catchment area population by the AB percentage, e.g. $230,000 \times 22\% = 50,600$. From local census figures, determine a typical client age group percentage, e.g. you might select 25–50-year-olds, which might be 45 per cent of the population. Multiply this figure by the catchment area AB population, e.g. $45\% \times 50,600 = 22,770$. This last figure represents your 'target' group.

Stage 3

Now all other things being equal, a 'target' group of 22,700 people could, on average, support some sixteen private practitioners. How many therapists are serving your catchment area? This is tricky, but you can adopt the following procedure:

- Get together a list of private practitioners operating within your own catchment area and any surrounding areas, together with their phone numbers and addresses. Many will advertise in the *Yellow Pages* and professional referral directories.

- On a suitable large-scale map mark the location of each practitioner, including yourself. Draw a catchment area for each practitioner. You will now have a series of overlapping areas. For each practitioner write down the proportion of their area that overlaps with your own, e.g. those who live on the boundary of your area may draw 50 per cent of their clients from your area. Those close to you may draw 80–90 per cent from your area. Those who are a mile or so outside may draw 30 per cent or so. Add together all the percentages and divide by 100.

This will give a rough indication of the number of practitioners competing for the same 'target' group of clients in your area. Compare this number with the number of practitioners you have already calculated your catchment area would, on average, support. This will give an indication of whether competition for clients is likely to be high or low.

This is not the whole story. Established private practitioners with a good reputation can draw clients from greater distances in the same way as out-of-town shopping centres can draw customers away from local shops. You may find that other private practitioners are specialising in different client groups from yourself. You may wish to consider contacting them to get an idea of how busy they are.

All of this is more important in the initial stages of planning and setting up your business. Once you start, you have already made a significant investment and you will find out soon enough if you have made a wise decision.

Assuming that you are satisfied there is sufficient potential demand for your services, you now have the problem of translating potential business into real business.

Step Four – Publicising your services

There is a Far Side cartoon by Gary Larson depicting aliens landing in a woodside clearing. Behind a tree is a man in a deerstalker carrying a rifle. The caption reads 'The aliens had landed on Earth to reveal to its inhabitants the mysteries of life and the universe, but they hadn't reckoned on Herb and his hunting rifle!'

It is remarkable how, sometimes, pioneering inventions or great works of art or music can remain undiscovered for centuries because their originator was not able to bring them into the public domain and receive the deserved recognition. Similarly, however good a therapist you may be, your expertise may not receive the recognition and reward it deserves unless you bring it to people's attention.

Advertising and publicity

For the purposes of a Business Plan you do not need to go into great detail. More on this and on marketing generally is covered in later sections. However, you should decide how potential clients are to be made aware of your existence and your services. It helps if you know your catchment area well.

The following is a list of possible actions you can take:

- Let as many people as possible know that you are starting a private practice. While you cannot counsel relatives or friends, their contacts might know people who may be potential clients.
- Take advice from other therapists and your supervisor as to the effectiveness of different forms of advertising.
- Put your name in relevant directories or registers. Remember that it may take a year before your advertisement appears in the new directory as such directories are usually only published once a year.
- Advertise in the *Yellow Pages* or *Thomson Local* telephone directories (see www.thomweb.co.uk).
- Advertise in the local newspapers and free press.
- Circulate details of your services to all medical and complementary health practitioners as well as healthfood stores.
- Circulate details to personnel managers in local authorities and organisations.
- Contact private hospitals, colleges, agencies and GP practices with a view to part-time or casual work.
- Give talks to local clubs and societies.
- Join any local branch of your professional organisation.
- Issue local press releases.
- Take part in discussions or phone-ins on local radio stations.
- Write articles for local magazines and newspapers.
- Produce an information leaflet about yourself and your services.
- Ensure you have business cards available to give to other professionals interested in your services.
- If you have a website, advertise yourself.

Some of these actions will cost money, and you will need to budget for this accordingly. For example:

Advertisements in directories and the media	£700
Postage	£80
Printing	£360
Telephone calls	£50
	£1,190

Step Five – Business objectives and financial planning

Unless you have other forms of income or intend to run your practice as a side-line, you need to plan and feel confident that your income will exceed your expenses, including personal living expenses, pension contributions, taxes and investment in your business.

It is easy to overlook this last requirement, but a frequent criticism of much of traditional British manufacturing is the failure to spend money on improving the skills of its workforce and their working methods and in replacing out-of-date and inefficient plant and equipment. Similarly, a therapist operating from a noisy, dingy consulting room, without the benefits of electronic equipment and systems and with no knowledge of recent effective therapeutic approaches, will be at a disadvantage.

Business objectives

For many new businesses, the first major objective is to reach a break-even point, i.e. when income and expenditure are in balance, before running out of money. Some never make it and, at the present time, many of the Internet-only companies, the so-called 'dot coms', are operating at a loss.

As a small business person, you should aim to have access to sufficient capital to last you well beyond your planned break-even point. One important purpose of a Business Plan can be to convince a bank manager, or whoever may make funds available, that you will be in profit and able to repay any loan within a reasonable time. How you do this is the subject of your short-term Business Plan objectives.

Short-term objectives

These are best illustrated by means of an example. Although the figures used are reasonably typical at the time of publication, they will be different for each person.

Suppose your objective is to break even within twelve months of starting the business. How do you plan, realistically, for this to happen?

Let us suppose you have done the previous exercises and satisfied yourself that there is sufficient potential demand for your services at the going fee rate, and that you are ready to move on to your advertising and publicity campaign. Let us also assume the following with regard to income and expenditure:

Income
You plan to charge £25 per hour. You anticipate about two clients per week to start with but rising to about twenty per week after twelve months. You intend to take a week off at Easter and Christmas and also the whole month of August.

Expenditure
One-off expenditures

Advertising and publicity initially	£1,190
Furnishing and equipping office	£4,000
Holidays in August	£750
Christmas	£150
Training courses in October	£300
Accountant's fees after 12 months	£150
	£6,540

Average monthly business expenditures

Office rent	£200
Motor and travel	£80
Gas, electricity, water	£80
Telephone	£40
Supervision and personal therapy	£70
Insurance	£20
Books and journals	£20
National Insurance contributions	£20
Stationery, postage, minor items	£20
Ongoing advertising	£20
Subscriptions	£10
	£580

Average monthly living expenses

Rent/mortgage, pension contributions (£100 per month), food, clothes, entertainment, household bills, etc.	£850
Total monthly expenses	£1,430

Now you convert all of this into a table. Assume you start in January, and project over two years.

Year 1

Month	Client sessions per month	Income (I) (£)	Expenditure (E) (£)	I – E	Cumulative surplus (+) or deficit (–) (£)
January	8	200	6,620	−6,420	−6,420
February	16	400	1,430	−1,030	−7,450
March	24	600	1,430	−830	−8,280
April	24	600	1,430	−830	−9,110
May	40	1,000	1,430	−430	−9,540
June	48	1,200	1,430	−230	−9,770
July	56	1,400	1,430	−30	−9,800
August	–	–	2,180	−2,180	−11,980
September	72	1,800	1,430	+370	−11,610
October	80	2,000	1,730	+270	−11,340
November	88	2,200	1,430	+770	−10,570
December	66	1,650	1,580	+70	−10,500
		13,050	23,550		

Year 2

Month	Client sessions per month	Income (I) (£)	Expenditure (E) (£)	I – E	Cumulative surplus (+) or deficit (–) (£)
January	88	2,200	1,430	+770	–9,730
February	88	2,200	1,580	+620	–9,110
March	88	2,200	1,430	+770	–8,340
April	66	1,650	1,430	+220	–8,120
May	88	2,200	1,430	+770	–7,350
June	88	2,200	1,430	+770	–6,580
July	88	2,200	1,430	+770	–5,810
August	–	–	2,180	–2,180	–7,990
September	88	2,200	1,430	+770	–7,220
October	88	2,200	1,730	+470	–6,750
November	88	2,200	1,430	+770	–5,980
December	66	1,650	1,580	+70	–5,910
		23,100	18,510		

Not an encouraging example! At this rate you would be in your fourth year before you recovered your initial investment. Furthermore, you need to have some £12,000 in capital to avoid bankruptcy in August of Year 1. Would a bank loan help? Perhaps you decide you need £12,000 to cover August in Year 1 and arrange to borrow this amount over two years with monthly repayments of £560. What would the first year look like now?

Year 1

Month	Income (I) (£)	Expenditure (E) (£)	I – E (£)	Capital left (£)
January	12,200	7,180	5,020	+5,020
February	400	1,990	–1,590	+3,430
March	600	1,990	–1,390	+2,040
April	600	1,990	–1,390	+650
May	1,000	1,990	–990	–340
June	1,200	1,990	–790	–1,130

There is no point in continuing. You are now bankrupt in May and are left owing the bank twenty repayments totalling some £11,000. You may lose your car if you have one and possibly your home if you have put it up as security against the loan.

Failure to calculate future cash flow and take action accordingly is a very common cause of bankruptcy. Now, it may well be possible to borrow a larger sum over a longer period, say £15,000 over five years, perhaps with a second mortgage. Again it would be essential to do a calculation along the lines shown above.

Note that although, technically, you were breaking even in the examples in the first year this was not enough to save the business unless you had sufficient capital of your own to see you past the point of maximum cash outflow.

At this point, you should be examining all of your income and expenditure to see if you can improve the viability of your business. For example, you may decide the following:

Income
Start to see clients before you go 'live', perhaps six per week in the evenings while remaining employed during the day. After twelve months of running the business and with extra training, raise fees to £30 per hour.

Expenditure
If possible, work from home and save £270 per month on rent, contents insurance and utilities bills. Put off pension contributions for two years or until you can afford them. Take only two weeks' holiday in August and at no extra cost. But continue with your training and personal development.

Now, what would the first year's picture look like? Your average monthly business expenditures have reduced to £310 per month from £580.

Your personal living expenses have reduced to £750 per month from £850 and your client base starts with eight clients rather than two.

Year 1

Month	Client sessions per month	Income (I) (£)	Expenditure (E) (£)	I – E	Cumulative surplus (+) or deficit (–) (£)
January	32	800	6,250	−5,450	−5,450
February	40	1,000	1,060	−60	−5,510
March	48	1,200	1,060	+140	−5,370
April	42	1,050	1,060	−10	−5,380
May	64	1,600	1,060	+540	−4,840
June	72	1,800	1,060	+740	−4,100
July	80	2,000	1,060	+940	−3,160
August	44	1,100	1,060	+40	−3,120
September	88	2,200	1,060	+1,140	−1,980
October	88	2,200	1,360	+840	−1,140
November	88	2,200	1,060	+1,140	
December	66	1,650	1,210	+440	+440
		18,800	18,360		

Clearly this is a much better situation. You have recovered your initial investment, and income will improve further with a higher fee rate. You have to meet your accountant's bill but this should not be a problem. However, tax rules do not allow you to count your living expenses as tax deductible. More on this later, but just to complete the picture, here is a rough tax calculation (note, the following assumes your set-up costs are all tax deductible, which may not be strictly correct):

Gross income	£18,800
Less set-up and business expenses	£9,360
(£5,190 + 12 × £310 + £300 + £150 (accountant))	
	£9,440
Less personal allowance (at time of writing)	£4,745
Taxable income	£4,695
Tax @ 10% on £1,960	£196
Tax @ 22% on £2,735	£602
Tax payable	£798

You should have no difficulty meeting an £800 tax bill that would probably be paid in two instalments.

As you should realise by now, short-term objectives are all about survival in the early stages of the business and cash flow is a crucial consideration.

Longer-term objectives

Although there are financial advantages to working from home, there are non-financial disadvantages, such as:

* Difficulty in separating work from home life.
* Insufficient space.
* Noise and potential disruption from other occupants.
* Difficulty in maintaining a professional environment and image.

One objective therefore may be to find a suitable office/consulting room. As a new private practitioner your fee rates will have to be competitive, since you have no reputation to justify anything more. However, you don't want to struggle to survive for years on end, seeing more clients than is good for you or for them.

A second objective may well be financial – to make sufficient surplus to keep client numbers at a manageable level, to invest in the business and your own personal development and to make pension contributions to permit a comfortable retirement.

A third objective may be to diversify away from a single business focus of seeing clients, to supervising other therapists, perhaps teaching and running courses or writing, all of these building on your own experience and expertise.

It is difficult at this stage to do realistic financial calculations extending over five years, say. However, let us suppose that, following the more successful version of your first year, you want to see what a second year might look like.

Year 2

Month	Client sessions per month	Income (I) (£) (@ £30 rate)	Expenditure (E) (£)	I – E (£)	Cumulative surplus (+) or deficit (–) (£)
					B/F +440
January	88	2,640	1,710[1]	+930	+1,370
February	88	2,640	1,060	+1,580	+2,950
March	88	2,640	1,060	+1,580	+4,530
April	66	1,980	1,060	+920	+5,450
May	88	2,640	1,060	+1,580	+7,030
June	88	2,640	1,460[2]	+1,180	+8,210
July	88	2,640	1,060	+1,580	+9,790
August	–	–	1,810[3]	–1,810	+7,980
September	88	2,640	1,060	+1,580	+9,560
October	88	2,640	1,360[4]	+1,280	+10,840
November	88	2,640	1,060	+1,580	+12,420
December	66	1,980	1,210[5]	+770	+13,190
		27,720	14,970		

Notes
1   Includes first tax instalment of £400 and accountant's fees of £250.
2   Includes second tax instalment of £400.
3   Includes cost of August holiday: £750.
4   Includes training course: £300.
5   Includes Christmas cost: £150.

It looks as if pension contributions are now affordable and, to make up for having made no contributions in Year 1, you could contribute, say, £200 per month. These are tax deductible provided the contributions do not exceed the allowed percentage of your profit, but the new stakeholder pensions do allow up to £300 per month (less 22 per cent contributed by the government), irrespective of earnings.

Can you afford an office and the associated bills? Probably yes. Another, say, £300 per month is affordable and also tax deductible. Of course, you will have a sizeable tax bill since your income is higher and your allowable expenditures are lower. For example:

Gross income	£27,720
Less business expenditure	£4,270
(12 × £310 + £250 + £300)	
	£23,450

Less personal allowance*	£4,745
Taxable income	£18,705
Tax @ 10% on £1,960	£196
Tax @ 22% on £16,745	£3,684
Tax payable*	£3,880

* When you read this, taxes will have changed, so you need to insert the current rates and allowances.

None the less, you do have the cash to pay your tax and, should you start making pension contributions and renting an office in Year 3, your tax would reduce by some £1,240 if your income remained at the above level.

Business administration

This is an often neglected but important part of any business. People, particularly politicians, tend to use the word 'bureaucracy' in a negative sense as if it was something undesirable and yet it is efficient bureaucracy that makes everything work. Answering telephones, dealing with correspondence and messages, keeping good records and files, ordering goods, keeping stocks, dealing with money matters, housekeeping, and organising things generally, all play a part.

As far as a Business Plan is concerned, perhaps the most important things to list are: the separation of your business bank account from your personal bank account; the method by which your clients pay; and how you intend to keep financial records and make provision for tax. We return to these matters later.

Summary of points for a Business Plan:

- Define the business you are (or intend to be) in.
- Define your resources.
- Define the potential demand for your services.
- Decide how you would publicise your services.
- Decide your business objectives and plan your finances.
- Decide the main aspects of your business administration.

Now, if you still want to continue, do your own Business Plan, show it to someone who is familiar with the concept and get some feedback. As mentioned earlier, banks offer an excellent service of vetting business plans. Would it be credible to someone in a position to lend you money? Even more important – is it credible to *you*?

> **Reflection issues**
> *   What are your business objectives? Are they realistic?
> *   What demand do you think there will be for your services?
> *   Does undertaking any of these exercises deter you? If so, what might that say about your attitude towards self-employment?

THE TYPE OF PRACTICE

In the previous section it was implicitly assumed that you are a one-person business, i.e. a sole trader and that you are operating the business full-time.

There are other options, which you might want to consider:

*   If you are in full-time employment, start a part-time practice in the evenings and weekends. There are many therapists who prefer to operate a small part-time practice and have no desire to become fully self-employed.
*   Find a part-time job that enables you to start a part-time practice during the non-employed hours or days.
*   Find guaranteed sessional work while developing your private practice, as this helps provide a regular income.
*   Join an existing practice or set up a practice with one or more other therapists.

You have already seen that it can be difficult to launch straight into a full-time practice from scratch. You have to spend money to set the practice up and it takes time to expand your client base to a level which recovers your initial investment and your business expenses, pays you a reasonable personal allowance and allows you to provide for tax, business and personal development and a pension.

If you have ready-made referral sources through previously established contacts then the work of publicising your services has already taken place and you probably could start full-time from scratch.

Otherwise, you do need sufficient capital to see you past the point of maximum cash outflow. In the first example given in the Business Plan this was some £12,000.

The alternatives

Continue in normal employment but utilise evenings and weekends to start a part-time practice

This is the most financially secure way of starting the business but you will need a lot of energy and probably an understanding partner.

A significant advantage is that you are testing the market and your fee level without undue risk. If the clients are forthcoming and judge that your services represent good value for money, you will begin to build a reputation and enjoy client loyalty. It also allows you time to get your name in the relevant directories, which you will need for advertisement purposes. If you reach the point where you are turning clients away and referring them elsewhere in a fairly short space of time, then you are either under-pricing your services or the time may have come to go full-time.

The income is not totally extra, though. You may well have to advertise your services and equip a spare room, possibly install an extra telephone line with an answerphone, and your extra income, less business expenditure, will be subject to tax.

If you are currently paying the standard rate of tax of 22 per cent, but your extra income, less allowable costs, takes you over the £28,400 p.a. taxable income threshold, then you will find yourself paying tax of 40 per cent on the excess. So don't go mad with the extra money.

The disadvantages of this option are that you could be working up to an extra ten to twelve hours per week. This will impact on any social or family life you may have enjoyed previously and probably affect your ability to carry out whatever share of household duties you were previously undertaking. An understanding partner, and/or understanding children, willing to give support, is very desirable and you may well need to have considerable discussion and agreement before you start.

Continue with a part-time job and utilise the non-employed hours or days to start a part-time practice

As before, this has the advantage of being relatively low risk financially and provides an opportunity to test the market and your own capabilities to run a business. It might be a suitable option for someone now released from previous family or other commitments. You will need to give consideration to the working hours of the part-time job and whether it is necessary or possible to renegotiate these. For example, you may need to release meaningful chunks of time in which to conduct a private practice, such as five half-days or two-and-a-half full days in a week.

Again, as before, your overall income should improve since you have more paid hours in the week, but your income tax liability will also increase almost immediately since your personal allowance and the 10 per cent tax band will probably have been used up in your part-time job. None the less, such an arrangement represents a viable option.

Find guaranteed sessional work to do alongside your developing practice

This is a similar option to the previous one and to the situation where you start a full-time practice with a useful base of clients already established. It has the effect of reducing the heavy cash outflow normally associated with starting a new business from scratch. You are, in effect, using paid employment or contract work to subsidise the development of your practice. As to where you find such work, this is for you to investigate. Frequently this kind of work is available where the organisation concerned does not have sufficient work to employ a full-time therapist or it does not want to employ at all, preferring a contractor whose services can be terminated at short notice without the penalties and on-costs associated with employment.

Alternatively, you may find a situation where there are practising therapists who cannot handle the peaks in workload.

Join or set up a practice with other therapists

This might seem a very tempting option. After all, if doctors, dentists, lawyers and accountants can do it, why not therapists? We are not referring to well-known agencies that train and employ therapists, but to private practices where each therapist is a partner in the business.

Clearly, there are advantages to being with other therapists. From a financial point of view, the renting and other costs associated with premises can be shared. It may be possible to employ a receptionist/administrator/bookkeeper to take the load off the therapists. It may also be possible to provide mutual cover at times of illness and holiday. Excess numbers of clients can be referred to other members of the practice. The practice may be able to offer a range of specialisms not possible for a single person. However, it would be prudent to have an agreed signed contract on how the practice will operate, including all the responsibilities of each therapist.

From a personal point of view, it would be possible to have a form of peer group supervision and professional support, particularly with difficult cases. None the less, the great majority of private practice therapists do operate as individuals and there are a number of reasons for this, including:

- The catchment area, particularly in sparsely populated rural areas, may provide only enough business for one individual.
- Clients may not wish to be switched between therapists. The relationship is intensely personal and takes time to develop with regular contact. With other professional groups, provided the individual is competent, it doesn't matter so much, and contact may be only once a year, or less, anyway.
- Individual therapists may prefer to have total control over their own businesses. Clients provide more than enough problems to occupy the individual therapist without the potential problems that may be generated by differences of opinion and behaviour between the practice's therapists. There could be arguments over how income and expenditure are to be shared, whether all partners are pulling their weight, how the practice should or should not be developed, and so on.
- From a legal point of view, the partners are generally all held to be responsible for all matters dealt with by the practice. Thus, malpractice of any type by one partner, if done in the name of the business, could involve all partners.

- Similarly, income tax on the profits made by the partnership can be claimed from any partner who may be left 'holding the baby'.

The choice of an option depends on individual circumstances, the location of a practice, personal preferences and finances. A choice is not irrevocable and for ever, and it may be that working with other therapists is a good choice until sufficient experience and confidence are acquired to go it alone.

FINANCE

In the many talks that one of the authors has given on private practice, financial matters don't seem to evoke the same interest and enthusiasm as other topics. No doubt, if all therapists had the unpaid services of a trained bookkeeper or accountant, the tasks of collecting fees, accounting for expenditure and generally helping to keep the practice on a sound financial footing would be very happily delegated. Unfortunately, this is not the case and even bookkeepers are obliged to make a living by charging for their services.

In any event, it does not pay to be too dependent on the services of others. A contact in the medical profession relied totally on her accountant and after a few years found herself owing the Inland Revenue a sum of £75,000 because the accountant had taken advantage of this dependency.

It might seem unfair, but if your accountant, your solicitor, your surveyor, your estate agent or even your GP or dentist gets it wrong, it is you that has to live with the consequences.

Keeping your finances in good order, though, is more a matter of self-discipline and common sense than one of financial expertise. So what's involved? (See Truman, 1977.)

Let us consider Mr Micawber's problem in Charles Dickens's *David Copperfield*:

Annual income	£1
Annual expenditure	19s 11¾d
Result	= Happiness!

Annual income	19s 11¾d
Annual expenditure	£1
Result	= Misery!

Fortunately for Mr Micawber, he and his hungry family were able to emigrate to Australia, where his wisdom and talents were rewarded.

The problem, which we have already met in the Business Plan section, is that of cash flow. If your expenditure exceeds your financial ability to pay then you are in debt, and if the problem persists you will be bankrupt and risk having your assets seized to pay off your creditors. Note that I used the term 'financial ability to pay' rather than 'income'. The term 'financial resources' could also be used. Nearly every business starts off by spending more money than it earns. A business survives this difficult period if:

1   it has sufficient capital of its own to see it through the period of negative cash flow (i.e. expenditure is greater than income)

or

2   it can borrow sufficient capital to do this

or

3   it can issue shares in exchange for sufficient capital.

Option 3 is not really applicable for a private practice unless it is turned into a company and complies with all the necessary requirements of company law.

    As a follow-up to the cash flow exercise undertaken in the Business Plan, let us consider the following case:

*   You borrow £15,000 over five years with monthly repayments of £375.
*   You start with eight client sessions in January at £25 per session, rising by eight sessions each month, except when you take holidays, where the income is reduced pro rata.
*   You spend an extra £500 in August on a two-week holiday in Year 1.
*   You also take a week off in April and in December of Year 1 and Year 2.
*   You spend £300 on training courses in October of Year 1 and Year 2.
*   You spend an extra £250 at Christmas in Year 1 and Year 2.
*   You get your office redecorated and re-carpeted in January of Year 2 at a cost of £1,000.
*   You take off the whole of August in Year 2 and spend an extra £1,000.
*   You pay your accountant's bill of £350 in February of Year 2.
*   You increase your fees to £30 per session for new clients only in January of Year 2.
*   Eight existing client sessions per month are replaced by eight new client sessions throughout Year 2 except as affected by holidays.
*   You do not exceed eighty-eight client sessions in a month. Your average business expenditure, excluding the loan repayments, is £600 per month (includes office rent of £200 per month).
*   Your personal allowance (known as drawings) is £900 per month (which includes £200 per month pension contribution in Year 2).
*   You have an additional start-up cost of £4,000 incurred in the first month.

Now do the following exercise! Lay out a table (which has been started off for you) as follows. Work out the cumulative cash flow (or bank balance) for the first twenty-four months. Do you make it or go under?

Year 1

Month	No. of client sessions	Income (£)	Business expenditure (£)	Loan repayment (£)	Drawings (£)	Total outgoings (£)	Cash flow (£)	Bank balance (£)
Jan	8	(15,000+) 200	4,600	375	900	5,875	+9,325	+9,325
Feb	16	400	600	375	900	1,875	−1,475	+7,850
Mar	24	600	600	375	900	1,875	−1,275	+6,575
Apr	24	600	600	375	900	1,875	−1,275	+5,300
May	40	1,000	600	375	900	1,875	−875	+4,425

When you have completed the table check it against the one shown. Don't worry if there are a few minor differences. No one can forecast this accurately anyway.

Year 1

Month	Income (£)	Business expenditure (£)	Loan repayment (£)	Drawings (£)	Total outgoings (£)	Cash flow (£)	Bank balance (£)
Jan	(15,000) + 200	4,600	375	900	5,875	+9,325	+9,325
Feb	400	600	375	900	1,875	−1,475	+7,850
March	600	600	375	900	1,875	−1,275	+6,575
April	600	600	375	900	1,875	−1,275	+5,300
May	1,000	600	375	900	1,875	−875	+4,425
June	1,200	600	375	900	1,875	−675	+3,750
July	1,400	600	375	900	1,875	−475	+3,275
Aug	800	600	375	1,400	2,375	−1,575	+1,700
Sept	1,800	600	375	900	1,875	−75	+1,625
Oct	2,000	900	375	900	2,175	−175	+1,450
Nov	2,200	600	375	900	1,875	+325	+1,775
Dec	1,650	600	375	1,150	2,125	−475	+1,300
	13,850	11,500	4,500	11,550			

Year 2

Month	Income (£)	Business expenditure (£)	Loan repayment (£)	Drawings (£)	Total outgoings (£)	Cash flow (£)	Bank balance (£)
Jan	2,240 [1]	1,600	375	900	2,875	−635	+665
Feb	2,280 [2]	950	375	900	2,225	+55	+720
March	2,320	600	375	900	1,875	+445	+1,165
April	1,770	600	375	900	1,875	−105	+1,060
May	2,400	600	375	900	1,875	+525	+1,585

Year 2 (*continued*)

Month	Income (£)	Business expenditure (£)	Loan repayment (£)	Drawings (£)	Total outgoings (£)	Cash flow (£)	Bank balance (£)
June	2,440	600	375	900	1,875	+565	+2,150
July	2,480	600	375	900	1,875	+605	+2,755
Aug	–	600	375	1,900	2,875	–2,875	–120
Sept	2,560	600	375	900	1,875	+685	+565
Oct	2,600	900	375	900	2,175	+425	+990
Nov	2,640	600	375	900	1,875	+765	+1,755
Dec	2,010	600	375	1,150	2,125	–115	+1,640
	25,740	8,850	4,500	12,050			

Notes
1   80 client sessions @ £25, 8 @ £30 = £2,240
2   72 client sessions @ £25, 16 @ £30 = £2,280

Comments

Although, technically, you run out of cash in August of Year 2, it is only by some £120 and this could be managed by deferring expenditures till September, borrowing from a friend, seeing a few more clients in June or July, etc. Alternatively, you may have an overdraft facility at the bank or be able to pay from your own resources.

You may notice that no provision has been made for tax. In Year 1 you just about break even as far as the tax inspector is concerned, since business expenditure of £11,500 added to loan interest of about £2,000 more or less balances your income of £13,850. It might in fact pay you to make your missing first year's pension contributions in January of Year 2 so that these can be offset against your Year 2's profit.

It is only when you do an exercise of this sort that you are able to foresee problems before they arrive. The last thing you need is an unauthorised overdraft, with the bank manager threatening to call in your loan.

Notice also the 'double whammy' of taking a holiday – no income but higher expenditure. No provision has been made for illness, but, to be on the safe side, you should perhaps budget for, say, two weeks' illness in the year when you are unable to see clients.

Again, we have assumed that your set-up expenses are tax deductible. (In reality, depending upon your situation, certain building costs and purchases may receive a capital allowance and are not tax deductible in the usual sense.) An accountant's advice would clarify this.

Having assured yourself that, on paper at least, you have a viable business, you now need to set up systems to monitor and control your finances. This is important. It won't work through optimism and wishful thinking alone.

Systems and administrative principles

We hope you don't shudder at these words. Some people do. But much is straight-forward and just requires the daily discipline to do it.

Separate business from personal finance

First of all, separate, as far as possible, your business income and expenditure from your personal income and expenditure. If you don't do this you will get into a dreadful mess and pay a heavy price when you come to year-end and have to submit your books and records for inspection by your auditor.

The easiest way of doing this is to keep a separate bank or building society account for all your business financial transactions. Of course, sometimes you have to pay cash out of your own pocket – taxis, parking fees, etc. – and sometimes you may use a personal credit or debit card. Always ask for and keep a receipt. It is easy to forget when you are just buying a dozen stamps, but it all adds up.

Day Book

Keep a Day Book (more on this later) where you record each item of income, the day received, who it was from, the cheque, number if paid by cheque, and the type of service paid for. In the same book, but on the facing page, record each item of expenditure. Use separate columns for cheque payments and cash or personal payments. Again, record the date, the cheque number, who the payment was made to and the type of expenditure, e.g. stationery, travel, office rent, etc.

At the end of each month, total up your income and expenditure. Work out roughly how much you can afford to pay yourself and how much you should put aside for the inevitable tax demand.

The Day Book logs your daily income and expenditure and is a primary source of data for your accounts.

Day Book: August 2000

| Income (left-hand page) | | | | | Expenditure (right-hand page) | | | | |
Date	Description	Type	Cheque no.	£	Date	Description	Cheque no.	Bank (£)	Cash (£)
1/8/00	J Jaques	client	0071	30.00	2/8/00	postage			4.39
1/8/00	S Jones	client	5641	30.00	3/8/00	gas bill	0091	26.20	
3/8/00	P Loi	client		30.00	3/8/00	Rymans	0092	34.99	
2/8/00	J Marie	client	0988	30.00	4/8/00	National Rail	0093	22.00	
4/8/00	P Jay	client	0911	30.00	4/8/00	stationery			5.30
		Totals					Totals		

Use a new page for each month.

Carry out reconciliation

Finally, carry out reconciliation. You can't do this until you have your monthly bank statement which may contain items not recorded in the Day Book, such as standing orders for National Insurance payments, direct debits, standing orders or pension contributions, and charges made or interest paid by the bank. This can be a tricky exercise and is covered later in detail.

Keep a separate record of expenditure by type

You will need a second and separate cash book in which to log all expenditures under appropriate headings, e.g. telephone and fax bills, motor and travel, advertising and publicity, etc. – you will need a book with, perhaps, twenty columns. It is best to enter all the details from your Day Book under the appropriate heading on a monthly basis. At year-end, total up all expenditures under each heading. Your accountant/auditor will need this to prepare your profit and loss account.

You can use a hardback book with about twenty columns extending over a double page to keep the expenditure record. It could look something like this but with more headings:

August 2000

Date	Item	Capital items	Premises costs (£)	Postage, stationery, etc. (£)	Travel & motor (£)	Total (£)
2/8	Postage			4.39		4.39
2/8	Gas bill		26.20			26.20
2/8	Stationery			34.99		34.99
4/8	Travel				22.00	22.00
4/8	Taxis				5.30	5.30
Total for August						
Brought forward July						
Carried forward September						

Start a new month on a new page.

Variations

If you have a good financial accounting package on your personal computer then you may need to enter data just once and usually the software will undertake reconciliation and throw out discrepancies for you to resolve. These systems can also work out the VAT payable too. However, do not expect perfection. The old saying 'garbage in, garbage out' (GIGO) applies to all computer systems.

Bank cheque or current accounts tend to pay very low interest rates, sometimes as little as 0.1 per cent, even on a balance of several thousand pounds. At the same time you will be charged a hefty fee if you overdraw on your business account without authorisation. A way around this is to make arrangements with the bank to have two accounts. The chequebook or paying-out account is used to receive all income and pay all expenditures, with a permanent balance being maintained of, say, £500. The other account, or paying-in account, holds all excess funds over £500 and tops up funds in the chequebook account and, more importantly, pays a more reasonable interest rate. Monitor this paying-in account carefully every month. Alternatively, you may have a chequebook account with a building society, but if you have a lot of transactions this may not be possible, since you are obviously running a business and involving the building society in the costs of processing your cheques and standing orders.

Fee collection

There is nothing to beat being paid on time; therefore we would advise that clients pay by cash or cheque at the end of each session. Monthly invoicing of private clients will inevitably mean that some clients will disappear owing you a month's money. You have to ask yourself whether your cash flow can take that risk.

Your views on this issue may well be coloured by your theoretical orientation and attitude towards the whole issue of payment. For some, the taking of money has a more therapeutic meaning than for others. However, regardless of therapeutic orientation, the matter of ensuring that payment is made is essential when your livelihood depends on being paid by your clients for the service you offer. Even when dealing with organisations that require an invoice, have the invoice prepared in advance and post it the same day. Your survival may depend on prompt payment. It can be helpful to check with the organisation in advance what payment policies are in place. Although you can encourage organisations to pay promptly, you cannot enforce payment. One local authority used to pay within thirty days as individual housing managers had control over payments. A change in policy meant that all monies were paid centrally and the payment time went from thirty to ninety days. No amount of telephone calls or letters speeded up the payment process. In addition, chasing payments requires time and energy. The reality in this case was that if you wanted the work you had to accept the payment terms and if you did not then someone else would.

You can outline your payment policy in your terms and conditions of business, which form part of your contract with the individual client or organisation. There is more about fees in Part Two.

Make provision every month for income tax

We recommend opening a separate tax saving account. Choose one with a good interest rate and reasonably quick access. Normally you will get a reasonable period of notice of how much tax you owe and by when it should be paid. This way, you won't be caught owing money you have not got and you will get interest as well – net of tax, of course. However, it is important to remember that due to changes in the taxation system tax is now paid ahead of time in two annual instalments, usually in January and July of each year (Whiteley, 2002). Inland Revenue staff are always prepared to help with any enquiries.

Systems and administration – some detail

Checking your bank statement(s)

Income

Pay the monies you receive into your business account via your paying-in book every few days. After entering all the details into your Day Book, write the name of the person and the amount on your paying-in stub, so that you can track the monies you have paid in, and write your account number on the back of all cheques being paid in. This way you reduce the possibility of cheques going astray. Normally the bank will credit your payments the same day, provided you bank before their close-off time, which might be 4 p.m. However, as you will be aware, you cannot draw cash against the cheques until they have 'cleared', which normally takes three to four working days, longer if you have an account with an ex-building society which uses the services of a clearing bank.

Checking your bank statement against your paying-in book is straightforward. Sometimes there will be differences. You may have forgotten to list all the cheques or you may have added them up incorrectly. Sort these out straight away. You may also have non-cheque income paid directly into your account, including bank interest. This form of payment is becoming more popular with a range of organisations and can be in your interest as it speeds up the payment process. You will come across the term BACS (Banks Automated Clearing System) which is the most popular form of this type of payment. It is usual for organisations paying this way to send you a note of the amount being paid and the date it is due to be paid into your bank account.

Expenditure

Your bank statement will generally not tally with the cheques you have written that month, for a number of reasons:

- Cheques you have written in previous months may not be presented or cleared until the present month.
- Cheques written in the current month may not be presented or cleared until future months.
- You may have a number of non-cheque items such as bank charges and standing orders or direct debits for items such as National Insurance, pension contributions, subscriptions, rent, utilities charges, etc.

As for income, check the validity of all entries when you get your statement. If you close off your books at the end of each month, make sure your bank gives you a statement for the same period. Banks try to spread production of statements to avoid the month-end peak, but if you are paying for their services there is no reason for you to go along with this. It is easier to reconcile your books and bank statements if there is a degree of consistency in the accounting period.

Keeping a record of expenditure by type

Just as a company keeps a separate account of its expenditures for raw materials, employee wages and salaries, rent and utilities costs, etc., so you will also need to do the same, but on a more simplified scale. Apart from being useful from a monitoring and control point of view, your accountant will need the information to prepare your profit and loss account and balance sheet for submission to the Inland Revenue and the assessment of your income tax liability. If you don't keep a record, your accountant will have to do it using your Day Book and bank statements and this will increase his/her charges.

Capital items

This covers all items that have a significant life, a significant cost and form part of the physical assets of the business, such as motorised transport, equipment (computers, fax machines, photocopiers, etc.), furniture and significant furnishings. These are kept separate because their cost is generally not 100 per cent allowable against profits in the year they were acquired, although there may be some exceptions.

With capital items, the cost is spread over the nominal life of the asset. For example, if you acquire a second-hand car for £5,000 for business purposes, this may be 'written down' or depreciated over five years, say, with £1,000 per year being charged to the costs of the business.

Note that the rules used do not represent reality. An asset may have a longer or shorter life in practice and it may have a residual value when it is disposed of. Your accountant will know the rules used by the Inland Revenue and be able to make the necessary adjustments.

Premises costs

This item covers rent, cleaning, repairs, redecoration and generally any work required to keep your business premises in good order. It also includes charges for gas, electricity and water and any rates or taxes levied on the premises.

If you are operating from a room in your home, then only a proportion of these costs are allowable, typically about a third. Again, an accountant's advice is helpful on this.

Postage, printing, stationery and minor office items and consumables

These items are self-explanatory.

Telephone and fax costs

These can include telephone charges for Internet use and the use of mobile phones as well as standard land lines. E-mail and text messaging via mobile phones are becoming increasingly popular and your overall costs can be quite substantial – £1,000 in a year would not be unusual. These costs are easier to justify if you have dedicated lines for business use. Otherwise, if your business shares a domestic line there is the problem of untangling business from personal or family use.

Publications and journals

All published material necessary to keep you up to date or to assist you directly in your business is an allowable expense.

Advertising, promotion and publicity

This would include advertisements in the *Yellow Pages*, *Thomson Local* directory, professional directories, newspapers and on the Internet; also the costs of any event used directly to promote your business.

Seminars and conferences

The cost of all activities, apart from basic training, designed to improve your professional competence.

Professional consultancy

It is a requirement for therapists to undergo supervision in order to retain their professional credentials and the fees involved are an allowable expense.

Professional subscriptions

The cost of belonging to all relevant associations, societies or organisations in connection with your business, including the costs of publications regularly subscribed to (avoid double counting these costs with seminars and conferences above).

Motor and travel

The costs of licensing, repairing, running, hiring and insuring any motorised vehicle used exclusively for your business (not the purchase cost which is a capital item). If the vehicle is also used for personal or social reasons, then only the business proportion is claimable as an expense. Other travel costs – plane, train, bus, taxi, hotel, etc. are also allowable.

Insurance

This includes professional indemnity insurance and your office contents insurance.

Bank charges

These are self-explanatory.

Accountants'/Auditors' fees

These are self-explanatory.

National Insurance contributions

These are a 'no choice' business expense but are *not* allowable for tax relief. Keep a record to balance the books.

Pension contributions

Strictly speaking, these are *not* a business expense but *are* allowable for tax relief (can you reconcile the logic with that for National Insurance?), subject to the age/net income percentages laid down by the Inland Revenue.

Drawings

Although not strictly a business expense, you should record all monies you pay yourself from the business, including money you put aside to provide for your income tax liability. Your accountant will also need the amount (though can probably deduce it) in preparing your balance sheet.

It is worth noting that your income tax liability, though, is not based on what you draw from the business (unlike a wage or salary) but on a calculated profit, i.e. business income minus business expenditure minus depreciation minus allowable pension contributions. So even if you drew nothing and lived on fresh air, you could still have a potential income tax liability. As Mark Twain wryly observed, 'In this life you can be certain of two things – that one day you will die and that there will be taxes.' In reality, your own personal income will be highly correlated with your profits unless you are either running down the business or making substantial investments in it.

Calculating your tax

At the end of each month you can use your Day Book entries to calculate your monthly income and expenditure, how much you can afford to pay yourself and how much to provide for tax.

For example:	£
Cheque income	1,530.00
Cash income	70.00
Direct payments into bank	425.00
Total income	2,025.00
Cheque expenditure (capital expenditure excluded)	321.21
Cash expenditure (capital expenditure included)	72.99
Direct debits and standing orders (excluding National Insurance, but including pension contributions)	256.34
Total expenditure	650.54
Notional profit	1,374.46
Less one-twelfth personal allowance of £4,745.00	395.42
Taxable income	979.04
Tax @ 10% on one-twelfth of £1,960.00 (163.33)	16.33
Tax @ 22% on residue (£979.04 – 163.33)	179.46
Provision for tax	195.79
Can pay myself (£1,374.46 – 195.79)	1,178.67

Although we have shown the calculation to the nearest penny, this is not necessary and at current tax rates it is probably simpler to put aside 20 per cent of your notional profit. It is your money and it does not hurt to over-provide and obtain some interest in the meantime.

You may also note that we have not included any capital expenditure in the calculation or any depreciation allowance arising from this. Again, this will result in an over-provision for tax but we imagine you would prefer to have more money in an interest-bearing tax account than is strictly needed. There is no problem in spending any excess once the taxman has been paid!

Other financial matters

Value Added Tax (VAT)

The current level of income at which you need to register for and to charge VAT is around £50,000 p.a. This level is not likely to be reached if you are just starting up your own private practice unless you are in partnership with others.

Considerable extra work is involved in keeping VAT records, and if you are obliged to charge VAT for your services at 17.5 per cent this means you either have to put your fees up, which can result in fewer clients, or else lose a proportion of your income in VAT.

Sometimes it is possible to reduce income to stay below the VATable level. For example, if you are travelling for your business on behalf of a client and the client pays directly for your rail ticket and hotel expenses, then you do not need to claim expenses, which will then not appear as income. This has no effect on your taxable profits.

Bad debts

Bad debts are more likely to arise when people pay by invoice rather than cash or cheque at the end of each session. If you are invoicing monthly, covering, say, four sessions at £25 per session, then £100 can be painful to lose. Failure to pay after a single session can be more readily contained, with the opportunity of discussion and, if necessary, amendment to the therapist/client contract. In theory, of course, there is the Small Claims Court, which, as part of the local county court, is fairly easy to find. You can obtain a claim form from this court. The Small Claims Court produces an excellent booklet on how to use the service and the staff are always willing to offer advice.

There could still be the problem of enforcing the court's judgement in what is a civil rather than a criminal case. You may not wish to employ bailiffs to hound a non-paying client, or to spend an undue amount of effort debt chasing.

In dealing with organisations you have little choice but to invoice them since you have probably agreed to do this as part of your contract with them. You may experience delays in being paid and you may need to remind them, but they are less likely to want to suffer the embarrassment of a court action.

The government has, somewhat belatedly, recognised the weaker bargaining position of the small company or trader and introduced legislation to curb late payers. Penalty interest of base rate plus 8 per cent is payable but, again, you may not wish to alienate the customer.

Keeping receipts

It is easy to forget to obtain or keep receipts, especially for relatively minor cash items such as postage, stationery, taxi fares, etc., but they all add up. If you do not have a receipt for any item you cannot claim it as a tax-deductible expense. The simplest method for keeping receipts is to keep them all in chronological order clipped together in a cash tin and at the end of the month staple them all together and place in a brown envelope, clearly marked on the outside with the month and year.

As already discussed, if you are thinking of setting up in private practice it is worth drawing up a Business Plan including a financial projection. It won't be matched exactly in reality but you will learn by doing it. As for day-to-day control, you need the discipline to keep all the necessary records until it becomes second nature. Remember, no one else will do it for you.

Reflection issues
- What type of practice is likely to suit you?
- Are you worried about the issues that were covered in this section?
- Which aspects of financial management do you feel less confident about and what actions do you need to take to strengthen your abilities?

MARKETING

Some aspects of marketing were discussed in the section on business planning, particularly market research and publicity and how you might be able to estimate whether there was sufficient demand for your services within the catchment area of your practice. Of course, the proof of the pudding is in the eating and you will find out soon enough if your estimates were realistic.

Marketing also overlaps with business planning and it is difficult to separate the two. For example, is your fee level a financial decision or a marketing decision? Some years ago, the top-selling luxury car in Venezuela was the Rolls Royce. Then the Cadillac overtook it. The reason was discovered to be the higher price of the Cadillac. Venezuelan oil millionaires liked to claim they owned the most expensive car available. The Rolls Royce dealer was quick to remedy this perceived fault and the situation was reversed.

Many hundreds, if not thousands, of books have been written about marketing, from the relatively easy-to-read guides on getting more customers to the almost unintelligible tomes on the mathematical modelling of advertising effectiveness.

In the section below, we set out the main components of marketing helpful to someone setting up or in the early stages of running a private practice.

Market research

You don't have to be a member of the Market Research Society to conduct some basic market research relevant to your business.

Know the area where you live and in particular your catchment area. Unless you are world famous, people won't be prepared to travel long distances to see you on a regular basis. Two of the authors practise in Blackheath, south-east London, and our catchment area typically extends up to three miles into the centre of London and up to ten miles in the direction of Kent. A typical travelling time by car is ten to thirty minutes; by public transport perhaps double this. However, as both of these authors also offer specialist services, there are clients who will travel from much further away to see them.

Clearly it is helpful if you are conveniently placed for public transport and car parking. Secondly, know your potential clients. An analysis of our own suggests:

Sex:	60 per cent female, 40 per cent male
Age range:	25–65, with most in the 30–60 range
Ethnic origin:	90 per cent white, 10 per cent black (mostly Afro-Caribbean)
Employment:	most in full-time employment – local government, education, health services, private sector, etc.; some self-employed; some not employed but supported by a partner
Car ownership:	about 80 per cent
Who pays:	80 per cent clients; 20 per cent employers, GP practices, partners, etc.

Your own clientele will differ from this profile but possibly not greatly.

Know your potential referral sources

Your clients will not materialise out of thin air. They need to know you exist, where you are, what you offer and how to contact you.

Unless you already have a good list of contacts you will need to advertise in one form or another.

When one of the authors started her practice the referrals were from:

Directories (*Yellow Pages*, BACP *Resources Directory*)	90 per cent
Other	10 per cent

As you become established, this pattern is likely to change and will be different for each practitioner. It could be any combination from the following sources:

- Direct advertising in directories and other media
- Personal recommendations
- Other therapists
- Local government
- Private organisations and service providers
- GPs

and so on.

Once you have started, make a record of how many clients come from the various referral sources and how much time and money you had to devote to each. This will help to determine the short-term cost effectiveness of each source; some sources may require a longer-term approach, involving a gradual build-up of your professional reputation, but in the end yield clients more suitable for your particular therapeutic approaches. It is also true that referral sources can change considerably.

In 1989 when Gladeana McMahon set up her full-time private practice there were only two therapists in the local *Yellow Pages* and advertising in this directory proved a lucrative source of referrals as she had a virtual monopoly. The competition included another co-author of this book, Stephen Palmer! However, for anyone starting out today in the same geographic area the situation is vastly different. There are over fifty people listed under the counselling heading alone, let alone the psychotherapy, stress management, hypnotherapy and psychology headings where there are many more.

Product range

Every business has a range of products or services, which it makes or supplies to its customers. Your business is no different. It is possible to be a specialist one-product business or service, like Coca-Cola or a heart transplant surgeon, but you will need a large catchment area to generate sufficient income.

In therapy, it is possible to specialise, with an approach for a particular condition or problem, but unless you have a widespread reputation you would need to be accessible to large centres of population.

In practice, it tends to be organisations which specialise, perhaps in employee assistance programmes (EAPs), HIV/AIDS, bereavement, victims of sexual abuse, couples, groups, women or young people. Perhaps they may confine themselves to a particular therapeutic approach, typically to that taught or supported by the employing organisation. Also, it is easier for an organisation to publicise itself than it is for a private practitioner. For example, if you can afford £500 to spend on publicity, an organisation employing twelve therapists could spend £3,000 and this would still be only £250 per therapist (known as the economy of scale).

Thus, most therapists are obliged to offer a general therapy service in the same way that GPs offer a general medical service. This is not to say that a few specialisms cannot be added to what you offer. You may find you have a particular rapport with certain types of clients (or they with you) or that you derive particular satisfaction or a sense of achievement from particular presenting problems. Every therapist is different.

Looking at the market, you may find that your catchment area contains, for example, farmers on the brink of bankruptcy, skilled workers being made redundant by dying industries, local government employees stressed by unreasonable demands made on them, or elderly people suffering bereavement or fearful of criminal attack. Each area will have its own profile of problems. The wealthy can suffer from drug abuse, alcoholism, suicide attempts and problems raising children. Again, it comes back to knowing your catchment area and its people.

When you are starting up your practice you may be anxious to generate sufficient clients to give you a reasonable income and be tempted to take on anyone, whoever they are and whatever the problem. This can be dangerous, particularly with unknown referrals where you may be concerned for your own personal safety, or in cases where your training has not given you the competence to provide successful assistance. It is also advisable not to have too many clients who require intensive long-term therapy. Otherwise, you will soon exhaust yourself and could suffer breakdown or burnout. In such cases it can be safer to refer on to other professionals who may have the additional capacity or knowledge to deal with them.

We cannot stress too strongly the importance of keeping your productive resources, i.e. yourself, in good health and good morale. Without these, both you and your clients will suffer.

Your products are non-standard and made to order rather than standard and supplied from stock, and this sort of business is always more difficult to manage since different blends of skills are required in each case and these are not necessarily obvious from an initial assessment.

In summary, what services you offer are personal to you. It is wise to take into account what you have been trained to do, what you are good at doing, what your preferences are and what the needs or desires of the potential clients in your catchment area are. You can extend your product range through further training but your productive capacity is limited by the number of client contact hours you can manage in a week. Use these hours to maximum effect.

Marketing is not just about promotion; it can also be a form of research. Remember promotion is just part of the marketing mix. The Chartered Institute of Marketing states that marketing is about satisfying customers' needs. It could therefore be helpful to put some of your marketing effort into an ongoing pro-gramme of research: for example, getting feedback via an evaluation form about the services you offer and how they could be improved, taking down details of how the person came to you. You could ask friends, family, ex-clients and other therapists about what trends and changes they see taking place, if any, over the next year, and try to understand future needs and how you can position yourself to meet these.

You need to build the concept of marketing into your thinking on a regular basis. For example, set yourself weekly or monthly targets. These could include contacting a set number of potential referral sources, or locating the most useful local branches of professional bodies where you can network, or contacting local groups where you can give a talk about counselling or a related matter. All these activities ensure that people know about you and the services you offer and, in turn, you also get to know about what is happening locally.

Advertising and publicity

There are two types of publicity that can be helpful: general publicity and personal publicity.

General publicity

First, there is publicity for counselling/psychotherapy itself, which, hopefully, is positive publicity. In recent times, such publicity has been mixed, with some journalists, writers or other public commentators attempting to rubbish 'talking therapies', either from lack of understanding, perhaps as a result of unproductive personal experiences themselves, or just because counselling/psychotherapy is an easy target.

It is difficult to prove scientifically that a course of therapy has resulted in positive measurable improvement which would not have taken place otherwise. Of course, there are studies that substantiate the way that various techniques can be successfully applied to various conditions. For some reason, the positive assertions of clients do not seem to be regarded as allowable evidence.

None the less, progress is being made and a recently conducted study by Professor King (Ward, 2000) does seem to have provided compelling evidence that, with regard to the treatment of depression, counselling achieved more positive results than GP care with its dependency on drugs.

Positive publicity of this sort generates a general increase in the demand for therapy, which can influence the demand for individual practitioners. This is rather like the way in which the opening of an attractive shopping centre can generate demand for the individual shops even though their own names may not have been explicitly advertised. Similarly, recognition of the convenience and usefulness of new technology equipment – personal computers, 'lap-tops', 'notebooks', 'diaries', Internet connections, mobile phones, etc. – has increased general demand without specific suppliers or brands becoming an automatic choice.

Where individual therapists are doing a good professional job, this fact is then spread by word of mouth and can influence such general publicity. However, it is really the domain of the professional organisations to promote the services of their members and, along with this, to set standards and encourage good practice. On the negative side, it requires only one or two highly publicised cases of malpractice to generate antagonism or cynicism.

Personal publicity

Secondly, there is publicity for you as an individual and your own services, and this is particularly relevant for private practitioners. How are potential clients to know that you exist and that you can help them?

We have already mentioned a number of methods in previous sections, but for a more comprehensive guide which covers the subject in more depth and variety I would recommend *How to Get More Clients* by Val Falloon (1992).

Of the wide variety of methods available, it is for you to choose and decide what sort of image you wish to project and to what sort of client. Cost can also be a significant factor, particularly with regard to mass advertising, which probably puts it out of reach for most people. It is interesting to note that, in advertising terms, a person has to see the name of a brand/person or product three times before it registers. If this is the case then placing one advertisement in your local paper is unlikely to bear fruit. However, placing a series of advertisements could prove expensive.

Follow-up

When you are starting up in business, how you respond to an initial enquiry, either from a potential client or from someone wishing to refer a client, is critical. An answerphone with a friendly yet professional message is essential. If you happen to be on holiday you need to change the message to '*the offices are now closed until* . . .'. Otherwise you need to respond quickly and positively to all queries. Some people have commented on the potential risks of such messages as it alerts people to the premises being unoccupied. This is certainly a risk. However, if you choose to become a self-employed private practitioner working from home it is not unreasonable to expect you to promote a professional image both for yourself and for the profession in general. We leave it to you to decide whether a telephone that is not answered promotes such a message.

Some therapists make arrangements with a local colleague to provide cover while they are away on holiday. This means incorporating an alternative name and contact number in your answerphone message. The advantages of this option are that you present a professional image to the person contacting you, your colleague covers for you and, of course, you can cover for your colleague when he or she is away. In addition, such cover can extend to existing clients who may be vulnerable and whom you have concerns about.

For new contacts it can be useful to send an information sheet about yourself, the services you offer, fees, practice address and how to find you by public transport or by car. This can help to turn most enquiries into live first visits as it provides the client with all the information they require. After that it is the quality of your service that counts.

If you are contemplating advertising, there are professional and ethical considerations to take into account. You cannot make extravagant claims about the efficiency of your services or about yourself (even if you believe them to be true), or about the benefits of your approach compared to others.

The British Association for Counselling and Psychotherapy (BACP) has provided guidelines for advertising. These include the fact that membership of BACP is not a qualification and it must not be used as if it were. In press advertisements and telephone directories, on business cards, letterheads, brass plates and plaques, etc., therapists should limit the information to name, relevant qualifications, address, telephone number, hours available, a listing of the services offered and fees charged and should not mention membership of the BACP unless they are accredited and/or a Fellow.

In oral statements, letters and pre-counselling leaflets issued to the public and potential clients, BACP membership may not be mentioned without a statement that it only means that the individual, and where appropriate the organisation, abides by the codes of ethics and practice and is subject to the complaints procedure of the British Association for Counselling and Psychotherapy. Copies of these codes and the complaints procedure are available from the BACP. In addition, all advertising and public statements should be accurate in every particular.

Also, practitioners should not display an affiliation with an organisation in a manner which falsely implies sponsorship or validation by that organisation. Any publicity material and all written and oral information should reflect accurately the nature of the service on offer and the relevant counselling training, qualifications and experience of the practitioner. In addition, the BACP believes that practitioners should take all reasonable steps to honour undertakings made in their pre-counselling information.

Image

Fundamentally, the image you project to actual and potential clients will come from your own image of yourself and your attitude to clients. This said, it can be hard to see ourselves as others see us.

By image, I don't mean the sort of manipulation of public perception undertaken by politicians and their spin-doctors in order to demonstrate their courage, wisdom and high moral standards. They probably need the spin, you don't.

There are a number of aspects to image.

Attitude and approach to client

There was a recent article in *Counselling and Psychotherapy Journal*, the journal of the British Association for Counselling and Psychotherapy, by a client who had had a number of therapists and was somewhat perplexed and disappointed by the results. She could see very little point in what the therapist was trying to achieve, if anything. Perhaps she is an isolated case, but we suspect not.

Clearly, our approach to a client is conditioned by our own training and experience. The authors subscribe to the belief that the approach used must be tailored to the needs of the client, rather than 'this is my approach, take it or leave it'. Not everyone may agree with this, but we have yet to find one single therapy that deals effectively with all clients and all client issues.

Many books have been written on the therapist/client relationship and this is not the place to add to their number. We only wish to say that the client must feel that he/she is in caring hands, and that this needs to be demonstrated both inside and outside the consultation as a fundamental part of your professional image.

Organisation and self-discipline

We have always been impressed by other people who keep their appointments on time, are pleased to see you, can remember your last conversation and can answer almost any relevant question either from memory or by an immediate reference to notes or books which are readily to hand. Such people convey an instant confidence that they know their business and have done their homework. The practitioner needs to consider in what ways these simple behaviours apply to them.

Dress and behaviour

How would you react to a therapist dressed shabbily or provocatively? Or to one who insisted on smoking in a small, unventilated room or who had an unpleasant body odour or reeked of a disagreeable perfume? Or one wearing or displaying symbols of their political or religious sympathies, which differed from your own? When did he last wash that shirt? When did she last visit the hairdresser? How can she afford all that expensive jewellery? These can be the sorts of thoughts that run through a client's mind and interfere with successful therapy.

Ask yourself what you would find distracting, sloppy, intimidating or otherwise in a therapist's dress or behaviour, and this will be a useful guide to your dress and behaviour. Ask yourself what you would find comfortable, reassuring and appropriate in your own therapist.

Environment

Although the consulting room environment is a major consideration, the rest of the premises seen or used by a client should not be ignored, or the immediate neighbourhood. A client is likely to absorb any amount of information about the therapist and draw conclusions as a result. It is in both of your interests that such influences are positive rather than negative. An excessively tidy environment could make a client feel that perhaps shoes should have been removed on entry. Similarly, an unswept path or unkempt garden with litter is unlikely to help. Corridors, waiting area, toilets, etc. do need to be kept clean, tidy, warm and attractive.

As for the consulting room itself, this should be consistent with the therapist and the therapy. The more analytical approaches may require a more formal, clinical, minimalist décor; a person-centred approach perhaps informal, warm and friendly furnishing. The therapist can, within reason, indulge preferences but care is needed to exclude items which could prove upsetting to a client – Christmas or birthday cards, family photographs, etc. could be painful reminders of what the therapist can enjoy but not the client.

Some therapists, understandably, are proud of their qualifications, as are many other professional people, and may wish to display framed certificates on the wall. There are differing views about the display of such items. Some people don't believe that it is necessary to impress or intimidate a client with such a display, believing that it is the application of knowledge and skills rather than their formal possession which counts.

Of course, the visual environment is not everything. Intrusive noise should be avoided, as should the possibility of being overheard by others. Smells can be cloaked by the use of subtle air fresheners. Seating should be comfortable enough to avoid fidgeting but not too comfortable to encourage either participant to doze off! You will find it helpful to locate a wall clock behind the client so that you can check the time and prepare for the session to close without obviously doing so.

Verbal and written communications

This aspect of marketing refers to communications that take place mainly outside the consultation sessions. It may start with a Client Information Sheet providing details about yourself, the services you offer and the terms and conditions under which you offer such services. It can also cover the length of sessions, their regularity and your fee structure. Such a sheet, well laid out, can be reassuring and helpful to a prospective client. Standard computer software such as Word or WordPerfect now mean it is possible to produce simple yet effective and professional-looking leaflets and information sheets.

The Client Information Sheet can contain the outline of the 'contract' between therapist and client or, alternatively, this could be a separate sheet given to the client and discussed at the first meeting.

Sometimes clients will make contact between sessions and frequently after the termination of a course of therapy. Apart from any therapeutic benefit it is good business practice to reply to everything as quickly as time will allow.

Telephone calls are common and will need to be fielded by an answerphone in the first instance. If you are working from your home you may wish to have two telephone numbers, one for personal use and the other for your business, as this allows you to prepare yourself for either a personal or a professional response. You may want to make a point of not disclosing your home telephone number, preferring to page your answerphone remotely at regular intervals. Otherwise, work is never finished and health can suffer. It can also save on your telephone bill if you can persuade the client to call you back. Twenty calls by you to a number of clients can be expensive. One call by a client is a more manageable cost.

Apart from a Client Information Sheet you are likely to need a letterhead and business cards and you may also find it helpful to invest in some compliments slips. All of these materials form part of your promotional strategy whether you are conscious of it or not.

How to get clients

We have already mentioned a variety of ways of marketing yourself. In addition, clients will also refer others to you and referral agents will too if they feel that you provide a good service. However, it takes time for word-of-mouth referrals to kick in as you have to see a lot of clients before this method brings results. You could also connect your therapy to a national campaign by looking at the benefits that your therapy offers and matching it to the issues of the campaign. For example, there are a number of established annual campaigns such as National Stop Smoking Day, National Stress Awareness Day or National Phobia Week. Creating your own website can also be used to attract clients (Harold, 2002).

Fees

The price of a product or a fee for a service is not just a financial decision but also a marketing one, for the following reasons:

- People expect a degree of consistency between the price of a product or service and their perceived value of its quality. The image of a product or service is more than just its content. The price of common commodities will vary from shop to shop but customers will not necessarily always patronise the cheapest. The reputation of the shop, the courtesy and help of assistants, the layout and décor and many other factors come into play to influence the decision to purchase.
- Rightly or wrongly, people tend to associate quality with price – 'you get what you pay for'. This is particularly true of highly paid professionals. If you are paying £250 per hour for legal advice you may well be more inclined to follow it than similar advice offered for nothing. People tend to be suspicious of an apparently good product or service offered at a knockdown price, thinking 'there must be something wrong with it' or 'where is the catch?'.
- There can also be a negative inference with a low-priced service that the provider him/herself does not value very highly the service being offered. You may have had clients well able to pay any level of fee attempt to bargain as a matter of principle. This can be a test of the value you put on your services, and your response may well be, 'I can refer you to others if you see my fees as a problem'.

Many therapists use a sliding fee scale to accommodate clients with differing abilities to pay. Others reserve one or two places for clients who can pay very little or nothing at all. One of the authors follows this latter route as she sees it as a way of giving something back to the community but in a way she can keep control of. Many practitioners find that a publicised sliding scale encourages too many people who can only afford the lower end of the scale to come forward. This can place the therapist in the difficult position of turning a person away, haggling about the price or taking on more clients than may be healthy in order to ensure the bills are paid.

Summary

Marketing is at the heart of all business. Taking it seriously means the difference between success and failure since the supply of counselling services takes place in a competitive customer-orientated market.

There are many aspects to marketing, as described in the sections above. Take the time to go through these again, one at a time, and assess your own business objectively. It is well worth the effort.

Reflection issues
- What aspects of market research apply to you?
- What basic materials do you require to get you started?
- What methods are you going to use to attract clients?

SECURITY AND CONFIDENTIALITY

We have already mentioned the need for clients to feel they are in a non-threatening environment. Small details can help – an outside light for evening clients, keeping pathways swept and free from ice, cutting back on large shrubs that could hide a potential mugger, etc.

Client confidentiality is important. If you schedule clients at intervals of an hour and a quarter this allows for a small over-run if necessary, as well as the making of notes, preparation for the next session and avoidance of clients meeting each other.

If you are working and there are other people in the same building, think about the measures you need to take to ensure that your conversations are not overheard or disturbed.

When you leave your consulting room make sure that no unauthorised people enter it and that client notes and records are securely locked away. Depending on where you are working, you might find it helpful to have a smaller, lockable, handheld metal filing system – available from main stationery stores – for current clients. Ex-clients' records could then be filed in a more traditional four-drawer lockable filing cabinet. If you are working from home you could store this cabinet in your garage. If you do this, it is essential that it is locked and/or that the garage is suitably alarmed and/or locked.

PREMISES

There are two main options when it comes to the choice of premises for a consulting room.

- Work from home.
- Rent suitable premises.

There are a number of advantages and disadvantages associated with each.

Working from home

For someone starting in private practice, this has the significant advantage of low cost. There *are* costs, of course, in particular the set-up cost of converting a suitable room, which may involve:

- the purchase of furniture
- purchase of equipment
- purchase of carpets, curtains, etc.
- redecoration

But, on an ongoing basis, costs will be marginal – extra heating and lighting, telephone charges, etc.

If the room is used exclusively for business purposes then there may be an additional charge in terms of business rates. This can be avoided if the room is also used for domestic purposes. However, if in doubt, check with your local authority for any regulations currently in force. Planning permission is not likely to be required unless the essential character of the house is changed, e.g. a large extension is built. There are, however, some disadvantages.

Unless you have a large house or genuinely spare room, which can be devoted to your business, it can be hard separating business from personal life. For many years one of the authors used a second bedroom as a consulting room but this involved clients walking through the living room. Her husband had to disappear and hide in the kitchen when clients arrived or left.

This worked well, but on two occasions he was discovered asleep on the living-room sofa, which caused some amusement to an understanding client, and on other occasions when a female friend was visiting or staying overnight they both had to squeeze up in a corner of the kitchen.

On another occasion, during a fairly intensive counselling session, there was a brief silence and the client and therapist heard a distinct snoring noise. Unbeknown to anyone, the cat had crept into the consulting room and hidden behind a sofa. It seemed that the therapeutic work held no interest for her.

We know of another example where the pet dog was allowed to stay in the counselling room during sessions. On one occasion, it took a dislike to a client and bit her. This is unacceptable behaviour since the counsellor was probably putting her own needs before those of her clients by allowing the dog to accompany her during sessions.

It can also be hard to disguise the smell of cooking which can permeate a small household.

There are many other examples where, because of the dual use of premises, disturbance or distraction can occur and detract from a professional image. None the less, when you are starting out this may be the only viable option.

Renting premises

Generally speaking, renting suitable premises enables you to tailor-make a room as a professional consulting room. It may come ready furnished, which, if the furniture is suitable, will save you having to buy any. You will need plenty of desk space and storage for telephone, computing equipment, books, files and stationery if you choose to do all your work from the office. Alternatively, you may decide to do your paperwork at home and simply use the premises to see clients. The décor can be of your own choosing, together with curtains, floor coverings, pictures and so on. The working environment is more controllable and you don't need to worry about other members of the family or pets.

Of course, whatever premises are chosen, location, safety and convenience for clients are still important. You would probably not choose premises on an industrial estate. A residential or residential/retail environment is more appropriate, as used typically by doctors or dentists.

The main disadvantage of renting premises is that of cost, where rent may be in the range of £200 to £500 per month – more if you aspire to Harley Street, less if you operate in a depressed or low-income area. You may have to agree to a tenancy of six or twelve months and pay a month's rent as a deposit as well as paying the rent in advance. The landlord could decide to repossess the premises (after giving due notice) or may be reluctant to carry out necessary repairs.

In short, if you intend to take out a tenancy on business premises you should exercise the same care as you (hopefully) would for a residential letting, and some legal advice would be helpful to clarify your rights.

Another alternative is to rent premises only by the hour or day, in which case you are likely to be sharing the same premises with others. This is generally a cheaper option than renting premises just by yourself, but it restricts what you can keep in the office and it also means that someone else is choosing the décor, etc. In this case, the letting agent is probably paying all the necessary bills and taxes, possibly contents insurance, cleaning, repairs, reception, etc., so you know exactly what your commitments are – just the hourly or daily rate.

A variation on this option is a straight sharing of premises with one other person, either with a joint tenancy (where you are both liable for the rent, utilities bills, council or business tax, and any damage), or with one of you being the tenant and sub-letting to the other. A landlord may be uneasy about this sort of arrangement as, with any agreement of this type, if one person leaves the landlord could be left with a potential squatter on his/her hands or a tenant who can't pay the rent.

Whichever option you choose, whether operating from home or from some form of rented premises, it is essential to know exactly what you are committing yourself to, whether you are complying with local authority regulations, and what legal liabilities you may be incurring, perhaps without realising.

Basic equipment needs

If you have sole or controlling use of your consulting room you can equip it as you see fit or are able to afford.

At a very basic level all that is needed is two, possibly three, comfortable chairs, window and floor coverings, space for storing client notes and details, a telephone answering machine and access to a toilet and wash-basin.

However, the constraints of such spartan furnishing will soon make themselves felt. A desk with writing surface, a high chair, drawers for stationery and writing materials, and cupboards or bookshelves for files, books and publications would perhaps be the next priority.

Then might come décor, including appropriate lighting, pictures, and perhaps a small table with a lamp. Finally, for an up-to-date working office, a personal computer, possibly with its own dedicated phone line, a printer, a scanner and a fax machine, preferably with its own line, though e-mail may render this unnecessary. Lots more storage space is needed for the 'mature' practice, particularly if the practitioner has diversified into writing or training. Training materials, professional journals and reference books can accumulate alarmingly.

There are many additions – facilities for tea or coffee making or storage of soft drinks; more electronic equipment in the form of portable laptop, notebook or palm computers, perhaps a zip drive for backing up files, etc.

Consideration also needs to be given to peripheral space – a clean, warm and tidy toilet with paper, towels, soap and air freshener; an attractive entrance and passageway, clean and in good decorative order; and storage space for cleaning materials and equipment.

Of course, for someone starting up it would be unwise to try to equip a consulting room with everything all at once, though in terms of potential space and storage it is worth looking to the longer term. A cramped office with no possible extra space or storage will soon become a real problem.

It is for the individual practitioner to set priorities for the acquisition of office items, furniture, furnishings and equipment. Cost, time saving and the creation of a pleasant environment may well be determining factors.

Insurance

As one of the authors was recently burgled, losing all her personal jewellery accumulated in the form of presents and heirlooms over many years, it was a relief to have a household contents insurance policy.

Naturally, insurance companies are in the business to make a profit and most of them do rather well. They can take their time over the settlement of claims and give the appearance of treating every claim as potentially fraudulent, which can add to the misery of genuine claimants suffering loss and disruption to their lives. None the less, they are a necessary, and sometimes legal, evil.

It is also important to remember that you need to check with your insurance company to see whether running your practice from home affects your contents policy. Some insurers will not cover you when you run a business from home, while others will place a restriction on the policy. This may state that the policy will only pay out if it can be proved that there has been forced entry. This kind of restriction is to clarify that clients may not leave the premises with your goods when they visit. There are now a number of insurers who provide specialist homeworker policies and it is worth investigating these.

If you are practising from rented premises you should also check what insurance is actually carried by the landlord; it may only cover accidental damage to the actual premises. It almost certainly won't cover any contents belonging to you and may not cover injury to third parties.

There is also indemnity insurance against professional negligence or malpractice. It is important that all private practice practitioners have suitable professional indemnity cover. Defending oneself, even if the case is found in favour of the practitioner, is a costly business, as well as one that can cause a considerable amount of emotional distress.

Illness or injury to a self-employed person can also have a devastating effect. No income is received but many personal and business expenses are still incurred. A few days are manageable but a few months could ruin your business, and what happens to your clients? When this happens, the differences between being employed and being self-employed can be appreciated – painfully. There is no six months on full pay and six months on half pay, or whatever employment conditions prevail. You are in deep trouble and the worry of losing your business can add to your problems and perhaps lead you to return before you are fully recovered. Again, this can be covered through appropriate insurance.

However, the downside of these policies can be the cost of contributions. It may prove more economical to keep a minimum of three months' money in a building society, earning interest, to be called upon should you be unable to work. Most bouts of illness that are likely to keep you from working are probably going to be of between one and six weeks and therefore a reserve fund of twelve weeks should be more than enough to provide the financial cover you will require.

Thus, there are several types of insurance that may well be applicable:

- building and contents
- public liability (accidents to third parties on your premises)
- professional indemnity
- illness/loss of earnings

For a full discussion of professional indemnity and the care and safety of clients, see Tim Bond's excellent book, *Standards and Ethics for Counselling in Action* (2000).

For insurance advice, use an insurance broker in whom you have confidence. Many professional bodies such as the British Association for Counselling and Psychotherapy and the British Psychological Society have links with preferred suppliers of such insurance.

Do not be afraid to shop around to get the best quotes. State clearly the services that you offer and the cover you are looking for. The onus is then on the insurance company to dispute this when you insure, and if they do not it makes it more difficult for them to wriggle out of paying subsequently.

RETIREMENT PLANNING

Just as you plan your career, so it is beneficial to plan your retirement, which these days can last as long as or longer than your career itself, particularly with early retirement at, say, 50 or so.

In planning for retirement, there are two main considerations. Will you have enough money to live comfortably and do the things you want to? What will you do with your permanent holiday?

An enormous amount of newsprint is devoted, particularly in the weekend papers, to all aspects of pension planning, personal investments, pitfalls, tax breaks, annuities, PEPs, TESSAs, ISAs and the like. This book is not the place to list every possible consideration or to make financial recommendations. However, for genuine independent advice, we would recommend *The Which Guide to an Active Retirement*, which covers virtually every topic relevant to retirement and planning for retirement. A new edition is brought out every year or so to keep up to date with the latest government legislation, regulations and schemes.

However, there are a few points worth making. The best time to start making provision for retirement is NOW (if you have not already started). The reason for this is the compounding effect of interest (or re-investment of dividends or returns), which can generate a large sum over a long period. For example: invest £3,000 in a cash ISA currently yielding 4.75 per cent tax free. If it were possible to leave this investment for years at the same tax-free rate of interest then it would grow as follows:

- After ten years £3,000 would turn into £4,731.
- After twenty years £3,000 would turn into £7,462.
- After thirty years £3,000 would turn into £11,767.
- After forty years £3,000 would turn into £18,559.

Of course, if it were possible to invest £3,000 every year under the same conditions the final sums would be much larger – £193,353 after thirty years and £343,121 after forty years – still significant sums of money and all yours, with no obligation to buy an annuity, though you could construct your own by living off the interest and prudent amounts of capital, and no charges by pension-providing companies to pay their administrative costs and shareholders either.

We are not necessarily recommending the above approach but a real and virtually risk-free return of 4.5 per cent is good, historically (6.5 per cent less 2 per cent inflation). The point of the above example is to illustrate the impact that regular savings can make over a long time. Providing for a pension does not necessarily mean signing up to an 'approved' pension scheme or pension provider.

The advantages of using a Treasury (or Inland Revenue) approved pension provider or scheme are:

1   You get tax relief (up to certain limits) on your contributions.
2   You don't have to do any work regarding investment choices.
3   The pension provider may (but not necessarily) know more about investments than you do.

The disadvantages are:

1   With a few exceptions, you cannot deal directly with the pension provider and if you do you still pay commission. You are obliged to use an agent who will take a generous commission – possibly the first year or so of your contributions. This is done, strangely, with the permission of the pension providers themselves who have threatened not to do business with those insurance brokers who wish to return a proportion of their commission to the customers.
2   Apart from the commission payable there are administrative charges every year that are not always declared up-front to the customer.
3   In 1997, the Chancellor of the Exchequer, in one of his renowned stealth taxes, removed the tax-exempt status of pension investments in equities (stocks and shares) by pension providers, thereby cutting the return payable to their customers.
4   Of the fund built up on your behalf, no more than 25 per cent can be taken as a tax-free lump sum on retirement (we will not go into the business of draw-down arrangements). The rest must be taken as an annuity (typically 7 to 8 per cent of the fund value at normal retirement age). When you die, any residual amount in the fund becomes the property of the pension provider.

Pension provision for self-employed people

A significant advantage to being employed by an employer who has a staff superannuation scheme is that the employer also makes contributions to your pension fund.

There is a range of options and possibilities:

1   This may seem strange but at the present time one of the best options is to repay capital off your mortgage, if you have one. Since tax relief is no longer available and special offers of discounted mortgage rates have a relatively short life you are likely to save more than if you invest in a cash ISA, typically about a 1 per cent advantage.
2   Make the most of any tax-free and charges-free investments, typically the last few years of any TESSA you took out before they closed in 1999 and the mini-cash ISA of up to £3,000 in any year.
3   As for specific pension provision, things are changing. Up to the time of writing only personal pensions have been available but these have been expensive with sales commission of 5 per cent or so and annual charges of 1–1.5 per cent, to

say nothing of the hidden and undeclared spread charges (the difference between buying and selling of units or stock). It has been calculated that most of the first year of your contributions can be swallowed up in this way, which is one reason why the UK's banking and insurance sector is so profitable.

4   The introduction of 'CAT' standards for ISAs and the new stakeholder pensions is designed to eliminate most of these charges. To meet a CAT standard for a maxi ISA of up to £7,000 invested in approved stocks, shares or bonds, charges cannot exceed 1 per cent. Similarly for stakeholder pensions, there are no up-front charges and a 1 per cent cap on annual charges. (How are the pension providers going to wriggle out of these constraints to protect their lucrative trade? Be sure they will try!)

5   With a stakeholder pension you can contribute up to £3,600 a year (£300 a month) even if you are not earning, so if you are feeling generous you could contribute to a non-earning partner's pension. (In fact you only need to contribute £2,808. The government contributes the remaining £792 (22 per cent of £3,600).)

6   As previously, the contribution limits for stakeholder pensions are as for personal pensions and dependent on age and income, as shown below:

Age	% of earnings contribution limit	Cash amount limit
Up to 35	17.5	£16,065
36–45	20	£18,360
46–50	25	£22,950
51–55	30	£27,540
56–60	35	£32,130
61 or over	40	£36,720

7   It is interesting to note that, at the present time (2005), widespread disillusion-ment with the whole pensions business, the low rates of return and exploitation by companies and the Chancellor of the Exchequer, has led many people to give up on pensions and put their savings elsewhere, e.g. in property. In many cases, this has proved to be a wise decision since property prices have enjoyed a ten-year boom. This is mostly as a result of low interest rates which make monthly repayments (the crucial decision factor) cheaper. However, no boom lasts for ever. There are risks and it is still possible to be caught in a 'negative equity' trap.

8   Possibly the best investment for the future is to invest in yourself and your business. Just as an employed person can earn more money through develop-ment of additional or improved skills and abilities and subsequent promotions, so the self-employed person can do the same by offering a more extensive or better quality range of products or services. So, take time to look at yourself and your business. A fee rate of £30.00 per hour will not permit much provision for savings or a pension. A fee rate of £60.00 per hour will permit significant provision.

9   There is a difference in the tax treatment of contributions for stakeholder pensions. Whereas, previously, a contribution of £100 attracted tax relief of 22 per cent or 40 per cent, reducing the effective cost to £78 or £60, for stakeholder contributions the government gives no tax relief but adds the relief at standard rate onto your contribution. So you pay £78, the government pays £22, totalling £100. If you pay tax at 40 per cent you have to apply for the additional 18 per cent relief on your tax assessment form.

Comments

It is a pity that successive governments have not acted like a prudent pension fund manager and invested your National Insurance contributions for your future pension, but they haven't. All income received by government goes into one big pot called the Consolidated Fund and is spent in the current year (somewhat irresponsible you might say). So when you get to retirement age, the government is relying on its income at that time to pay your state pension. With a rapidly growing ageing population, the taxation burden on earners and companies to fund an acceptable level of state pension would become intolerable – hence the various tax breaks and concessions to encourage personal pensions and saving and reduce dependency on the modest state provision. Some countries do it differently, loading extra costs on to employers (e.g. France, Germany) to subsidise higher state pensions, but this then reduces their competitiveness, which is one reason why there is pressure on EU governments for taxation harmonisation.

With state provision at a low level and likely to remain so, your own savings for the future will probably determine your standard of living on retirement. The earlier you start to put money aside, the better, and it is sensible to take advantage of any tax concessions available.

As a test, sit down now and work out what your income is likely to be in retirement, preferably in real terms, i.e. after inflation. Will you still have a mortgage or other commitments to meet? You will probably need an income of at least half of what you are getting at present to maintain a reasonable standard of living. Do the sums and take action now. Make arrangements for a standing order at your bank so that you don't see the money you are saving and are not tempted to spend it. When you get more income, increase your standing order accordingly.

Other considerations

People who have been used to a daily routine of paid work can find retirement unsettling. Whereas, before, weekends and holidays were to be treasured, looked forward to and enjoyed, suddenly all days become the same. Every day is a holiday; how can that be when days turn into weeks, months and years? Some lose a sense of purpose, direction and status, not realising how daily contacts with others can give a sense of fulfilment or achievement. Ordinary work pressures – to turn up on time, look presentable, behave properly, organise oneself and one's work, perhaps please a boss and get praise – all of these disappear. For many people, the work ethic has become a powerful learned habit and, without it, they don't know what to do.

In a number of ways, self-employed people are better able to cope with retirement since work discipline comes from within rather than being externally imposed by an employer. You have the choice of working twenty hours, forty hours or sixty hours in a week or even none at all. You can, up to a point, vary the type of work you do – direct counselling can give way to training, supervising or writing. You can restrict yourself to certain types of client where your own approach works particularly well or where you obtain personal satisfaction in your achievements. If you have the money, you can take extended leave or holiday. You can attend courses to develop your knowledge or skills in areas of interest.

None the less, it is an unusual person who wants to work until disability, illness or death dictate otherwise.

As mentioned previously, it is possible to draw a pension from your own pension fund from the age of 50. Of course, the benefits would be much less than if you retired at 60, 65 or later, since the fund has to cover you for more years, possibly thirty or fifty rather than fifteen or twenty. Even so, it is an option, particularly if you have made substantial pension provision or put aside savings beforehand. Perhaps the mortgage has been paid off and children are self-supporting, so financial commitments are much reduced.

It is not an objective of this book to tell you what to do when you retire. This is very much a matter of personal preference. However, it is important to give it some thought and planning. Retirement can be broken down into four aspects – the four 'F's:

Finances   (what most of this section has been about)
Family and Friends (the opportunity to strengthen relationships)
Fitness   (to maximise your retirement years)
Fun   (the chance to do what you really enjoy doing)

All of these are important. You can start to lay the foundations now.

PART TWO

The professional skills

In this section we will be looking at running your practice in an efficient and knowledge-based way so that you do not run into difficulties with practical issues if and when they arise. You will only be required to deal with some of these aspects on a regular basis, some occasionally, and others, hopefully, never. However, you do need to know what your legal obligations are, and how to protect both your client and yourself, if the need arises. Make it a regular habit to at least look at the contents page of professional journals that land on your doorstep – it may well be that some new piece of legislation which might affect you is being summarised.

LEGAL REQUIREMENTS

Perhaps we are fortunate in the UK in so far as we do not yet have a culture of litigation enthusiastically aided and abetted by lawyers. However, the situation is changing, as one can see from TV advertisements for 'no win, no fee' claims and 'where's there's blame, there may be a claim', etc. (What these adverts do not say is what proportion of any payout is taken by the lawyers and others!)

In addition, when you accept money to undertake a task such as therapy in private practice, the various laws protecting the consumer come into play. If you work for an agency, in either a paid or voluntary capacity, then the agency affords considerable protection if claims are brought. There is still a need for each individual to act with 'due care' towards others. However, the agency is likely to have its own cover to protect those working there. When you are a private practitioner, taking money for your services, the law will presume that you are working in a professional capacity and have the skills required to do so. If a claim is made, it will be made against the individual practitioner.

We will start by looking at some of the legal requirements for self-employed therapists and some of the equally 'grey' areas that fall under this heading (Jenkins, 2002).

Confidentiality and the law

Therapists normally go out of their way to stress the confidential nature of their services to clients – the exemption usually cited being 'danger to self or others'. However, in reality, no one bar a solicitor or barrister has the right to total confidentiality – not even doctors. The law can demand far more from practitioners – you can be subpoenaed for reasons including court action, potentially dangerous clients, and professional impropriety. It is therefore important to be aware of what information you may be required to share, and in what circumstances, so that you can prepare your administration and note-taking with this in mind.

Courts of law may require to see a therapist's notes and/or any material that is related to the client: for example, tapes, questionnaires, letters, drawings, etc. (Palmer, 2002). While it is extremely unlikely that you would find yourself in this position, you need to bear this possibility in mind, as it is likely to affect such matters as the content of your note-taking.

If you work, either regularly or occasionally, with young people and you consider it likely that some abuse (of any kind) is involved, you should also be aware of the Children Act 1989. Reporting child abuse is not mandatory in England and Wales, but most professionals will be obliged to act on suspected abuse under the terms of their professional Code of Ethics and in line with the concept of a Duty of Care. Where a person under 18 confides information regarding harm that has been done to them, e.g. rape, then you may be obliged to take the matter further – informing the police or appropriate agency. This can create ethical difficulties for the therapist.

When you are in private practice you do not have colleagues to discuss these matters with or an agency policy to guide you. Although it is likely that you would discuss the issue with your supervisor, your professional association and perhaps your professional indemnity insurance provider, the actual decision-making lies totally with you.

This is a further example of where your case notes may be required to substantiate the facts of a situation. As a self-employed therapist, you are not obliged by law to reveal such evidence unless a court order is taken out requiring you to submit it. In addition, it would be helpful for you to think about your policy regarding confidentiality in advance of any such difficulties arising.

It is only possible to cover a limited number of aspects relating to therapy and the law in this book and we would strongly recommend that you read further on the subject. You will find a list of recommended reading at the end of the book.

Taping

Many therapists ask about taping sessions. Some are students on courses where examples of client work on tape are a requirement of the course; others like to use taping as a way of looking back at specific sessions, taking tapes to supervision. Indeed, in cognitive-behavioural therapy it is considered good practice and the norm to tape sessions. Others like to give the tape to the client as a way of offering them the opportunity of listening to the work again if they so wish. Provided the client (as well as the agency, if appropriate) agrees to the taping of sessions, there is no problem.

However, there are considerations. These tapes could be requested in a court of law, and precedent means you would have to submit them if asked to do so. Beyond this, you need to consider where you could keep such tapes safely, how long you would wish to keep them for, and possibly inform the client of these decisions. If you do not give clients a copy of their own taped session, how would you feel if a client asked to receive a copy of a tape? Would this concern you?

Do remember that it is your responsibility to be aware of any changes the government might make to the laws of confidentiality and access. Relevant professional journals will usually provide you with such information, or at least alert you to such changes, and this is where belonging to a professional body becomes helpful.

Fees

You may be wondering, as a new practitioner, what level of fee to charge. As mentioned in Part One, in its simplest terms, your scale of fees will depend on supply and demand. The BACP publish an annual *Counselling and Psychotherapy Resources Directory* and you can request a copy for your area (as well as nationally, if you wish). The therapists listed will normally quote their fees or fee scales, and this will give you a better idea of what would be appropriate for you. Bear in mind the following. Unless you are very anxious to build up a clientele at all costs, don't pitch your fees too low. Apart from the volume of clients you will then need to see to make a reasonable income, you will also have the difficulty of raising fees when the demand for your services becomes greater.

As a rule, try not to adjust your fees too often, or have too many fee scales. It will make life more complex for your record-keeping, and, even within the bounds of tight confidentiality, it is always possible that your clients may know each other and accidentally discover that they pay different rates for your services. Where you decide to increase your rates, do this for new clients only. Allow existing clients to remain on the agreed rate – with the exception of long-term clients (say, of two years or more) where it would obviously be appropriate and expected that the fees should rise somewhat over time.

Review your fees annually and state this as a clear policy on the Client Information Sheet you give to all new clients. If you do not do so it could be argued that any increase in fees changes the initial contract, whereas by simply stating 'fees are subject to annual review' you will have covered yourself should you wish to raise your fees. It is helpful to be aware of the current charges of other therapists, if you are in a competitive environment.

Payment of fees

The simplest way of receiving payment is on a session-by-session basis. This ensures that your record-keeping and cash flow are up to date, and that you are not wasting time chasing money or working with bad debt. You can give the client a receipt for their payment (simple receipt books can be purchased in any good stationery suppliers) and keep a copy for yourself. This protects you from queries regarding over- or under-payments.

However, some of your clients may prefer to pay against an invoice, and you will need to offer this facility if requested. It may be that some clients come to you through work or private health insurance schemes, and you may be asked to bill the insurer directly. You do not necessarily have to do this: you have the option of asking your client to make the claim against your invoice to him, while he pays you directly. This has the advantage that you are paid more quickly, and leaves the client to chase his insurance company if it is tardy about payment. In such cases, your invoice will need to be more substantial in terms of its presentation – listing full details of who you are, your qualifications and practice location, together with exactly what therapy you have offered, dates, times, length of sessions, etc.

Some clients also prefer to be billed periodically, and – unless you have any strong views to the contrary – provided you believe the client to be trustworthy and unlikely to default, this should be an option that you offer.

There are some therapists who operate a 'deposit' scheme, where one session is always paid for ahead of time, thus discouraging the client from 'no shows' and ensuring that the therapist does not lose a session payment in such cases. Some people may feel that such a scheme puts the financial aspect of therapy too high on the agenda and that it is better, as with all businesses, to build the possibility of some bad debt into your overall income predictions. However, should you have difficulty with unpaid fees, and if all reasonable requests for payment are ignored, going through your local Small Claims Court (see p. 77) is a simple procedure. In all probability the mention of possible legal action will persuade your client to settle his account.

If you do decide to take this course of action you will need to send the client a letter stating that if you do not receive payment by a certain date you will take legal action. Send the letter by registered post so that you have evidence of posting and, if the client does not pay by the stated date, all you need to do is decide whether to follow through or not. We suspect theoretical orientation will colour your view of the various options open to you.

Contracts

A contract between therapist and client ensures that both parties are clear about the services offered and the individual responsibilities of each party. Keenan (1995) defines the first essential element of a contract as being the offer of something and its acceptance. Thus, the offer of counselling and its acceptance is the counselling contract.

Eric Berne (1966), the founder of Transactional Analysis, defines three different levels of contract – the administrative, the professional and the psychological. While primarily looking at the administrative, or business, contract, which deals with the practical arrangements and agreements, Berne also identifies the professional contract as embracing the focus of the counselling and how it will proceed. The psychological element concerns the unspoken, and often unconscious, expectations that are brought to therapy by the client – and/or the therapist. For the purposes of this book we are concerned with the administrative contract.

When a client gives you money for your services, this contract is legally binding. So what are the critical, 'not to be missed' elements of a reasonable contract between client and therapist? Is a verbal contract adequate? If written, how lengthy can it be before your client becomes too confused and anxious about it?

A verbal contract is just as legally binding as a written one – but much harder to remember and prove with regard to content, should it come to that. It is also asking a lot of a client at their first session to expect them to remember everything that rolls off your tongue expertly because you have done it so many times before. Therefore, a written contract makes much more sense for you both.

Take time to decide what you wish to put in your contract, and review it regularly to ensure it represents your current practice. Circumstances are sure to arise which you had not expected and you will need to build these in as your experience increases. Share this information with your client and agree the elements of the contract, ensuring that the client understands those sections that are not open for negotiation.

If you have produced a Client Information Sheet, this will contain all the information regarding the terms and conditions under which therapy is offered. The information sheet can be sent to the client together with a covering letter confirming the time of the appointment before they attend for the first session. By doing this you ensure that the client has the relevant information about what is expected of both parties. In addition, it shortens the contracting process when the client attends for his or her first session.

Some therapists prefer to work on the contract together, allowing the client to take a copy away following the first session in order to read it through again and ask any questions. Some therapists like to provide a contract which is 'cast in concrete', simply asking the client to agree to the terms and conditions outlined.

A sample Client Information Sheet is shown below.

Amy Helper
11 Anywhere Street, Anywhere, London SE9 TNR
Tel. 020 8841 4712. Fax: 020 8841 2009.
E-mail: **amyhelper@anywhere.com**

CLIENT INFORMATION SHEET

Training

I hold an MSc in Counselling and a Diploma in Integrative Counselling and I also engage in a minimum of 30 hours' Continued Professional Development annually.

Accreditation

I am a Senior Registered Practitioner/Accredited Therapist with the British Association for Counselling and Psychotherapy (BACP).

Experience

I have been fully self-employed since 1995 and work as a Counsellor and Psychotherapist. I started my counselling work in 1985 and have worked in a variety of commercial, local authority and medical settings. I receive referrals from a number of sources including general practitioners.

Codes of ethics

I adhere to the BACP Ethics for Counselling and Psychotherapy.

Fees

If you wish to cancel an appointment I require a **minimum of 24 hours' notice**, otherwise you will be liable for the full cost of the missed session. Payment by an individual (cash or cheque) is made at the end of each session. Organisations are invoiced on a monthly basis or at the end of a given contract period. Fees are subject to annual review and non-payment of fees may result in legal action being taken.

Supervision

Good therapeutic practice requires that the regular supervision of cases is undertaken. Supervision can be seen as a form of quality control and a way of ensuring that therapeutic standards are maintained.

Confidentiality and access to case notes

The trust between client and therapist is crucial to the success of the therapeutic process and I treat all information disclosed as confidential. Any details my Supervisor receives are also treated as confidential and we do not disclose client details to any third party without the client's permission. However, if in my opinion a client is either a danger to himself or herself or to others I do reserve the right to inform appropriate agencies. In addition, confidentiality can only be offered within accepted legal boundaries. It is my practice wherever possible to inform the client first should confidentiality need to be breached. I keep brief notes on our work together which you are entitled to see at any time if you so wish.

Therapeutic process

I offer prospective clients an Assessment Interview. This gives both of us the opportunity of considering whether we wish to work together. It is just as important that you feel comfortable with your therapist, as it is that your therapist feels able to work with you. If we decide to work together we would arrange to meet for an agreed number of sessions.

There is no obligation to attend all the sessions arranged and you are free to terminate your therapy at any time. A review session will take place at the end of the agreed number of sessions and this is where we jointly assess progress and what further action, if any, may be needed. If we decide at the Assessment Interview not to work together I am usually able to provide details of alternative therapists or agencies.

Sessions last for one hour and if you are late arriving we still terminate at the usual time so as not to delay the next person. I leave 15 minutes between sessions to allow those people wishing to remain anonymous the opportunity of doing so. I see clients (Monday to Friday only) during the day as well as in the evening.

Contact

There are times when I am unavailable for various reasons. To allow messages to get through I have a confidential voicemail service that I encourage clients to use when I am not personally available. If I need to contact you I simply leave my name and telephone number should you be unavailable.

How can counselling or psychotherapy help you?

A therapist or psychotherapist aims to help you gain a perspective about whatever is troubling you. Together we identify what might be stopping you from reaching your full potential and what action you need to take to improve your situation.

Therapists are trained to look beyond presenting problems to possible underlying causes. The aim of the therapeutic process is to help you understand and accept yourself, to change your behaviour to that which is more productive for you and to help you move towards becoming the kind of person you want to be.

My approach

There are many different models of therapy to choose from. I work integratively as I do not believe there is one model of counselling or psychotherapy that helps everyone, as each person is an individual and what might suit one person may not necessarily suit another. I aim to be sensitive to the cultural and ethnic origins of individuals and to people's religious beliefs and sexual orientation. I operate my practice along the lines normally associated with an equal opportunities employer.

Fee scale

Individuals
Assessment Counselling Interview £45
Per session £45

Couples
Assessment Counselling Interview £60
Per session £60

A minimum of 24 hours' notice is required for cancelled appointments, otherwise the full fee is payable.

Travelling instructions
National Rail:	Anywhere Station
Buses:	54, 89, 75, 108
Parking:	parking spaces usually available outside the premises

Some therapists may wonder if an information sheet and the subsequent contracting process are off-putting to the client in any way. However, it is the view of the authors that the boundaries and security that it offers the client, as well as the sense of professionalism and care it projects, far outweigh these concerns.

It is important for the therapist to refer to the contract and to go through its contents in a way that inspires a sense of 'working together', rather than simply reading out a list of rules. How you work through the contract with your client can also add to the therapeutic process.

While clients need to know about such issues as confidentiality, session times and fees by the start of the first session, everything else can wait until the assessment or first session ends.

If you are to work together you can then complete the contracting process by asking your client to fill in a Client Details Form. Once this has been done not only does it provide useful contact details but it also acts as evidence that your client has read, understood and agreed to the terms and conditions outlined.

A sample Client Details Form is shown opposite.

Whether you ask only the client to sign the contract – or you both sign it – is a personal issue.

CLIENT DETAILS FORM

Personal details

Surname: _____

Given names: _____

Address: _____

_____

_____

Post code: _____

Tel. no(s):   (Home):_____ (Work): _____

Mobile: _____   Pager: _____

E-mail: _____

Date of birth: _____

How did you get to hear of me?_____

(e.g. friend, doctor, *Yellow Pages*)

Doctor's details

Name: _____

Address: _____

_____

_____

Post code: _____ Tel. no.: _____

My signature below confirms that I have read and understood all the information detailed in the Client Information Sheet supplied to me and that I agree to abide by the terms and conditions outlined therein. In addition, I also give my permission for Amy Helper to make contact with the appropriate external agencies if she believes I am a danger either to myself or to others.

Signed: _____

Date: _____

Right to practise – professional expectations

At present there is no legislation to prevent anyone setting up as a therapist. However, in reality, if you do wish to develop a stable and reputable practice, there is a variety of professional expectations that clients will either assume or ask about, and you need to be able to adequately meet these expectations as you build up your practice.

Palmer and Szymanska (1994) suggest checks that a (potential) client should consider and these are listed below. You might like to consider how you would respond to these, and whether there are any gaps in your expertise relating to your clients' expectations. There may be other items you would want to add to this list.

In the experience of the authors, including a copy of such information with the Client Information Sheet promotes a sense of professionalism on behalf of the therapist. Clients seem to like having an information sheet, as this helps them understand what they are letting themselves in for before attending for therapy, and also a sheet that outlines the 'dos' and 'don'ts' in terms of professional expectations.

ISSUES FOR THE CLIENT TO CONSIDER

1   Here is a list of topics or questions you may wish to raise when attending your initial Assessment Counselling Interview:
   a.   Check your therapist has the relevant qualifications and experience.
   b.   Check the approach the therapist uses, and how it relates to your problem.
   c.   Check that the therapist is in Counselling Supervision (a professional requirement).
   d.   Check that the therapist or counselling agency is a member of a professional body and abides by a code of ethics. Wherever possible obtain a copy.
   e.   Discuss your expectations of counselling and the goals you want to achieve.
   f.   Ask about fees (if your income is low check to see if the therapist operates a sliding scale) and discuss the frequency and estimated duration of counselling.
   g.   Arrange regular review sessions with your therapist to evaluate your progress.
   h.   Do not be coerced into a long-term counselling contract unless you are satisfied that it is necessary and beneficial to you.

If you do not have a chance to discuss the above points during your first session, discuss them at the next possible opportunity.

GENERAL ISSUES

2   Therapist self-disclosure can be therapeutically useful. However, if sessions

are dominated by the therapist discussing his/her own problems at length, raise this in the counselling session.

3   If you feel uncomfortable, undermined or manipulated at any time within the session, discuss this with the therapist. It is easier to resolve issues as and when they arise.

4   It is unethical for a therapist to engage in sexual activity with current clients and research has shown it is not beneficial for clients to have sexual contact with their therapist.

5   Do not accept gifts from your therapist. This does not apply to relevant therapeutic material.

6   Do not accept social invitations from your therapist. However, this does not apply to relevant therapeutic assignments such as being accompanied by your therapist into a situation to help you overcome a phobia.

7   If your therapist proposes a change in venue without good reason (e.g. from a centre to the therapist's home), do not agree.

8   If you have any doubts about the counselling you are receiving, discuss them with your therapist. If you are still uncertain, seek advice.

9   You have the right to terminate counselling at any time you wish.

(adapted from Palmer and Szymanska, 1994)

Continuous professional development will be a part of any good, accredited (or non-accredited) therapist's planning, and expanding your skills should include continually building upon general basic expectations for professional counselling.

Using the Small Claims Court

While you will hopefully not incur bad debts – or, at least, not too many of them – you will need to decide how far you wish to pursue them if and when they arise. One way of doing so, as mentioned earlier, is through the Small Claims Court. The first advantage of taking this route is that, quite probably, once your client has been informed that you are proceeding in this way, they will settle the bill and save themselves a lot of further aggravation. The second is that it is fairly cost-free, because solicitors will not be involved.

The small claims track is designed to provide a procedure whereby claims of not more than £5,000 in value can be dealt with quickly, and at minimal cost to the parties involved. The intention is to make the procedure as simple as possible, without any need to call on solicitors. The reason for this is that the costs that can be recovered by a successful party are extremely limited, and it is therefore considered uneconomic for solicitors to represent the parties in a small claim. You will be given clear directions as to what paperwork you need to supply, and the hearing itself will be very informal – and, if all parties agree, the court can deal with the claim without a hearing at all. In other words, a court could make a decision based on the statements of the case and documents submitted, without your having to turn up to give oral evidence.

As mentioned above, the costs which can be recovered in a small claims case are limited, and include only fixed costs attributable to issuing the claim, any court fees paid, travelling expenses and – importantly for you – loss of earnings.

Some therapists are concerned that taking a client to a Small Claims Court would be a break of confidentiality. However, this is where the Client Information Sheet comes into its own, as it states that 'non-payment of fees may result in legal action being taken'.

Producing reports and attending court

Apart from the Small Claims Court, it is also possible that you may find yourself required to attend court as an expert witness on behalf of a therapy client. This is a very rare occurrence, so don't sweat over it, but you should at least be prepared for the possibility (Palmer, 2002).

In what circumstances might you be asked to attend court?

As a therapist in private practice it is unlikely – although not impossible – that you will be working with clients who are being prosecuted on any account (where you might be asked to provide evidence of their character, or of criminal offences confided to you during therapy). You are more likely to be asked to act as a witness in a case where, for example, your client is involved in an insurance claim of some sort. Within this category, the most common would be some type of accident – for example, where your client is suffering from post-traumatic stress disorder and is suing for damages. In such a case, you might be asked to provide evidence (not alone, but in partnership with medical experts) that would demonstrate whether the accident had affected the client's ability to lead a 'normal' life. It is probable here that the client will actually request your involvement, thus avoiding the moral dilemma of whether or not to offer it.

Other possible reasons for attending court might be client suicide, professional negligence, or – though extremely unlikely – prosecution for assault, fraud or some other serious offence.

With regard to written evidence, you may have an option of producing your case notes, or writing a report to encompass the work you have done with the client. Where you have a choice, report writing will, while being more time consuming, be a clearer form of presentation (unless you have the most immaculate case notes). You may well be able to charge a fee for this report, so do not omit to check.

Your report should contain the following:

1   An introduction which includes details of yourself and – briefly – your background and qualifications, i.e. you will need to state your competence to act as a witness.
2   A brief history of your client's situation, how he was referred to you, when you started working with him, and how often you see him.

3   Your initial assessment of the client (if this has not already been submitted by someone else) and your subsequent plan of treatment for him.
4   How treatment has progressed, and what eventual goal/outcome you are working towards and hoping to achieve.
5   Your view on whatever is relevant to your client's claim – e.g. his ability to return to work as a bus driver after being involved in a serious car accident – will also be important. It is vital to stress, however, that this is your informed opinion only, and you would not be asked to support such testimony alone – medical, psychiatric and occupational therapy reports would also be requested in such circumstances.

You may have to present your written report in court. When doing so, do not assume that the court has read the report ahead of time, even though you will have submitted it earlier on. Where there are key areas of the report that you wish to highlight, practise beforehand, speaking slowly and clearly so as to be certain that the important points are emphasised. Evidence always needs to be stated in the clearest terms to ensure that it is not 'missed' or misinterpreted.

You should be given clear instructions prior to the case as to how to present yourself, where and when. You will also, almost certainly, be working with a solicitor at this stage, representing your client (or yourself), who will also give you guidance. Where this is the first time that you have appeared as an expert witness, your barrister will usually guide you through the best way to present your evidence, and any pitfalls to avoid, ahead of time.

Here are some further points that may be helpful as the hearing approaches:

•   On the day of the hearing, you may find your client's barrister with little spare time for questions, so try to obtain answers to any queries ahead of this.
•   Ask if there is a Witness Support Programme at the court, to explain the procedures to you prior to the case.
•   Where a barrister is representing the client, his solicitor, while attending the hearing, is not allowed to speak in the court (which is why you may see notes being passed back and forth).
•   As a witness, you will be asked to wait outside the court until called, while the case is going on.
•   In practical terms, you will increase your confidence by dressing smartly and acting professionally (speaking slowly and clearly and considering your answers carefully). Be aware, as well, of your non-verbal communication. This will add to the weight of the statements you make.
•   The order of proceedings for you as a witness will be that you will first be questioned (under oath) by the barrister calling on you as a witness. You will then be cross-examined by the other side's barrister. Finally, you may be questioned again by the first barrister.
•   Where your term in the witness box is interrupted by any sort of adjournment

– say, a break for lunch – you must not speak to your legal team at all. You may feel a little as though you have been 'sent to Coventry', but it is essential, and you may only speak to them after your testimony is complete.

• Finally, where court attendance is mandatory, you may need to block off flexible periods of time. Courts are notorious for delays and postpone-ments, so, when you are given a date for the hearing, be prepared for this to change.

Additional record-keeping (e.g. storage, letters, ethical systems)

We have already discussed the various types of client documentation you may keep and this section takes a look at ensuring the safety of these documents, both currently in use and where therapy has terminated.

First and foremost, make yourself familiar with the stipulations in the Data Protection Act. This was most recently updated in 1998, and checking the present regulations, as well as keeping abreast of any further changes, can be done by logging on to www.dataprotection.gov.uk. The Data Protection Registrar is usually very helpful and in an attempt to make the process as simple as possible will complete your form for you so that all you have to do is check it and pay the £37 annual registration fee.

You will also need to abide by the rules laid down by your professional association for confidential document storage. The BACP can provide you with a range of fact sheets to assist you.

In legal terms, professional Codes of Practice are not necessarily recognised in a court of law. While they do carry some weight in some courts, it is important to ensure that you adhere to the Data Protection Act. However, from an ethical point of view, where you agree to work within the code of ethics and practice of your professional body, you will need to adhere to the guidelines laid out by them, in addition to, and where they are not in conflict with, the Data Protection Act.

The important point to keep in mind, therefore, is that these ethical requirements do not necessarily fully cover your legal requirements. You are under further obligation to ensure that you fulfil these as well, in case of investigation.

So what constitutes 'safe-keeping' in relation to written notes and other documentation?

There are two main considerations:

1   Physical safe-keeping of records (against fire or theft, for example).
2   Confidential safe-keeping of records (against their being read, or otherwise used, by third parties).

Physical safe-keeping is likely to take the form of a locked cabinet, and you need to think about where you keep the keys and the need for a second set just in case the first set is lost. These must also be kept confidentially, somewhere known only to you (and hidden well enough not to be 'stumbled across' by anyone else) and one other named person.

It is quite common, if your private practice is run from your home, to consider the garage, if you have one, as useful storage space – which, indeed, it is. However, you will need to think about the security aspect of this, as mentioned earlier. Many of us store quite valuable items in our garages, and yet it can be one of the easiest parts of our home for a thief to break into. While it is unlikely that counselling files would be of interest, it is still ethically important for you to ensure that they are, again, locked away, with key(s) in a safe, confidential place. As mentioned earlier, you could use a small portable lockable system in the office for current clients and a standard lockable four-drawer filing cabinet in the garage for ex-clients.

What would happen to your files if you were not there? Who else knows where you keep your files? While, on the one hand, you are encouraged to be as discreet as possible with regard to their physical whereabouts, on the other hand, should anything happen to you, someone else must be able to 'rescue' these files and ensure their destruction or safe-keeping. Your supervisor would be an ideal person to give this information to. Give him or her written instructions as to where your files are kept, where the keys are kept, and to whom he or she may reveal this information in order to ensure their care.

It would not be realistic to expect your supervisor to physically deal with this him/herself, but your supervisor should not be unhappy about notifying someone trustworthy, and advising them on how to act. This person would, in agreement with you, take care of all matters pertaining to your clients and client work should an accident befall you. In addition, if you were dead it would relieve those who love you from having to deal with such matters at a time of emotional difficulty. Even if you felt they were willing to undertake such a task, it is unlikely that they would be aware of what would be required if they were not in the same line of work.

If you live with a partner, it goes without saying that he or she needs to know who to make contact with in such circumstances. If you live alone, then you may need to alert a family member or keep a note on you to alert the authorities to the job that you do and the need to ring your supervisor so that he or she can take care of your clients.

It might also be helpful to give your supervisor a regularly updated list of the telephone numbers of your current clients. Again, should you be involved in an accident, you may need someone you can trust to make urgent contact with clients in order to inform them of this. Your supervisor may be willing to take on this responsibility, as it is an unlikely event. However, it does give peace of mind. It also means that someone has access to client contact details without having access to the content of their files. To bring this round 'full circle' you may also wish to keep a note of your supervisor's telephone number to hand – mobile phones are ideal for storage of these details – so that he or she could be contacted and alerted in such an instance. If you live on your own, you may wish, if your supervisor is agreeable, to leave a spare key with him/her just in case.

Many therapists will now be using computer storage systems, or at least considering this. As you will note from the Data Protection Act 1998, you must have your client's permission in order to store records in this way, and they have a right to ask to see such information. While we cannot imagine a circumstance where a therapist working ethically and with integrity would not allow his client the option of seeing his case notes, it is as well to bear this fact in mind. It is also worth thinking about what needs to be done with any client information stored on your computer, and your supervisor or named executor needs to have information about *all* of the material he or she will need to take care of.

Human error, such as failing to lock the cabinet, or accidentally leaving a file on view, means it is important that you take care to ensure that you do not leave clients' personal details – name and contact address, telephone number, etc. – in the same place as your case notes.

Use a code for each client on the case notes file, and keep a separate folder (or card index file) that lists his or her personal details and links them to the case notes. It is a similar principle to keeping your bank card pin number in a different place from the card, and it goes without saying that this list also must be kept under lock and key, or otherwise securely stored.

Regarding the retention of client files, there is no particular law or legal requirement that specifies the exact period for keeping these files. However, the Law Society recommends that a period of six years plus one year (for safety) after the last therapeutic contact with the client is a good benchmark. The BACP also supports this, as six years is the time limit within which a client is able to use the complaints procedure. It is also recommended that, where a client is under 18, their records be kept until they come of legal age.

After this period, you may get rid of the files. At this point we would suggest the following:

1   Consider keeping your client's initial assessment sheet 'just in case' you wish to refer to it for any reason.
2   If you have access to a shredder, shred everything else to ensure efficient and complete disposal. If not, then you could burn the notes to ensure they cannot be accidentally read by anyone else.

As you progress, you will devise your own best practice for storage of papers and your ethical and legal responsibility in relation to this, which will be dependent on your working environment and the system you personally find the most efficient and valuable.

Reflection issues
- What further information do you think you need in order to feel confident in running your practice?
- What type of contracting process do you want to put in place and what paperwork do you require?
- Are the recommendations made in this book excessive or necessary?

COMPETENCY

Minimum training requirements

Currently anyone who wishes to can set up as a therapist, place an advertisement in a newspaper publicising their services, and wait for the clientele to arrive. The only drawback to this (apart from any personal conscience on the part of the 'therapist') is that it under-estimates the increasing knowledge base of the general public as to what therapy involves, and what qualifications they should seek before committing themselves to a particular therapist.

While therapy training is a basic requisite for good practice, there is debate about what constitutes a minimum training standard. Current lack of regulation of courses can mean that some are set up purely in order to increase fees brought into the college, without particular care given to the quality of the course.

While it is not a necessity for a therapist in private practice to be accredited by a professional organisation, it is a sensible ambition. We believe it provides a recognised standard by which the therapist is evaluated and one that clients recognise and have confidence in. In addition, you may wish to expand your self-employed therapy activities to encompass such additions as lecturing, training, supervision, and so on, and a professional accreditation will enhance your prospects of getting this extra work.

It therefore makes sense when starting out to elect to train on a course that the BACP has accredited. This makes the path towards BACP accreditation much easier. The *BACP Training Directory* lists over 500 organisations offering courses.

Many – perhaps the majority – of therapists reading this will already have qualifications at least to diploma level, and the question can then become, what further training should I be considering?

There are several considerations here. First, are you considering gaining accreditation by a professional body? If so, check out the minimum study period required, and consider whether you have enough theory under your belt to meet that requirement, or whether you need more. Second, have you taken an integrated course but now wish to specialise, for example, in Transactional Analysis? In this case, further specialised study will not only increase your knowledge and skills, but also enhance your credentials to work in this area.

Third, consider how you will plan your continuous professional development (CPD). Accreditation by any professional body will require you to undertake CPD (the BACP, for example, currently require thirty hours per annum) and you can make the choice between short (one- or two-day) courses, and more substantial further training.

Fourth, how much time can you give to further study when you are in a work situation and possibly trying to develop a new business? Many colleges will offer specialised training over a certain number of weekends or evenings per year, to enable you to continue studying at the same time as working. The *BACP Training Directory* is an excellent source of course and college information.

Before committing to specialisation, read and research the pros and cons of the different models in relation to the client 'market' you are working with, or considering working with. Do you wish to work long-term or short-term? With children and young people especially? Are there certain client groups that appeal to you, e.g. the bereaved, the elderly, drug and/or alcohol agencies? If so, discover the therapy models more widely used with these groups, contact agencies for their views and experiences and read books.

If you are thinking of setting up in private practice it is the opinion of the authors that the minimum qualification required to practise is a diploma and that the therapist should also consider the issue of experience. In private practice anyone can make an appointment. Unless you are very clear in stating that you only work in a particular way with particular clients, the likelihood is that you will see a wide variety of clients and client problems. To be able to feel reasonably confident in dealing with such a wide range of clientele, the more experience you have the better.

Until recently one of the authors has made it a policy to undertake one certificated training course in therapy or a related area annually. This has not only helped with increasing therapist knowledge and ability to help clients but it has also added to the credibility of the therapist in terms of perceived capability by clients and others.

The role of personal therapy

While not universally mandatory, some professional bodies and counselling agencies do insist on the therapist being in personal therapy as part of their ongoing CPD. So up to a point it is a personal decision. We have spoken with therapists who consider it essential to good practice, and others who feel it is an expensive 'add-on' that they could do without. The majority of therapy courses usually insist on a certain number of personal therapy hours to complete the course. This requirement does make sense – if for no other reason than the importance of seeing and learning from counselling in action, and understanding what being a client feels like.

Once qualified, it usually becomes more of a personal or theoretical issue – especially when you are self-employed. Some theoretical orientations encourage therapists to continue in personal therapy while they are working with clients, and this can mean for many years. Is it just another unnecessary cost to the practice? Or is it something you should not do without?

Evaluation and auditing of the practice

In simple terms, evaluation and auditing means accounting for what you do and why you do it. If you have previously worked in a counselling agency or similar environment, you may be familiar with the term 'audit'. For agency funding to continue, the providers of the funding usually require evidence that the therapy is 'working', i.e. that, by whatever form of evaluation it has been decided to use, positive client outcomes can be shown. The term now commonly used in these instances is evidence-based practice.

As a therapist in private practice, your obligation to provide evidence of your CPD will usually be limited to your professional association. Beyond this, you do not need to measure and evaluate positive client outcomes except on your own behalf. However, professional accountability is important if you want to ensure that your practice is successful.

In private practice, accounting can take many forms:

- Reviewing your own ongoing development as a therapist.
- Ensuring that your qualifications are up to date and sufficient for the work that you undertake.
- Continually ensuring that your practice is run in a professional and cost-efficient manner.
- Inviting client feedback either formally or informally as a measure of the success of their therapy.
- Monitoring statistics of the number of sessions per client against the problems they bring.
- Using supervision as a 'quality control' mechanism.

Your professional association is likely to ensure that you set measurable criteria for your professional development. For example, BACP Accredited Counsellors are required to undertake thirty hours of CPD annually to keep accredited status. In addition, the association will also keep you informed about professional standards and new qualifications.

Ensuring that your practice is run in a professional manner can either be an ongoing task, or based on an annual 'competency audit' where you review your procedures for running your practice generally. Such an audit could include record-keeping systems, IT use, marketing, finances, evaluation of skills, etc.

For either of these self-evaluation processes, it will be important to set yourself goals so that you know at the start of the year what you hope to achieve by the end of it. You may then find it helpful to break these targets down into smaller goals, to be reached within shorter time periods – say, six months, a month, or even a week.

This gives you the opportunity to constantly review whether you are 'on track', or need to re-evaluate and re-set your goals. Make sure that your goals are written down, clearly, on the left-hand side of a sheet of paper, or in a notebook. On the right-hand side of the paper, write down the action that you need to take in order to achieve that goal. For example, if you write down 'Increase number of clients', 'Work shorter hours', 'Improve record-keeping', alongside this you must write down exactly what you need to do and how you plan to achieve this and by when.

It obviously makes sense, if you wish to develop your practice, to find out from clients what works and what does not work.

Counselling agencies tend to use systems such as the CORE model to make inventories of the clients' progress through therapy and statistically interpret outcomes. While this does indeed work well, it might be beyond the needs and purposes of a private practitioner, given the time and effort such a model would take. What you really need to know, in order to constantly develop best practice, is laid out in the sample Client Evaluation Questionnaire shown below.

CLIENT EVALUATION QUESTIONNAIRE

Your views are very important in helping me monitor the quality of the counselling work I undertake. Any information you provide will be treated as confidential.

Using a scale of 0–8 (0 = very poor and 8 = excellent) please rate the following.

Pre-Counselling Contact

1   How well was your initial enquiry dealt with?
     (e.g. efficiency, helpfulness, etc.)

     0   1   2   3   4   5   6   7   8

2   How useful did you find the Client Information sent to you?

     0   1   2   3   4   5   6   7   8

The Counselling Environment

1   How would you rate counselling facilities offered?
     (e.g. counselling room, parking facilities, etc.)

     0   1   2   3   4   5   6   7   8

The Therapist

1   How helpful did you find your therapist?
     (e.g. understanding, approachable, skilled, etc.)

     0   1   2   3   4   5   6   7   8

2   What did the therapist do that you found most helpful?

_____

_____

3   Was there anything your therapist could have done differently that would have been more helpful?

_____

_____

Your Progress

Using the rating scale 0–8 (0 = 'feeling awful', 8 = 'feeling good') please rate the following.

1   At the beginning of your counselling how would you have rated yourself?

0   1   2   3   4   5   6   7   8

2   After the counselling how would you rate yourself?

0   1   2   3   4   5   6   7   8

3   What did you find most helpful about the counselling offered to you?

_____

_____

Any Other Comments

Thank you for taking the time to complete this questionnaire. Please return in the s.a.e. provided to: Amy Helper, 11 Anywhere Street, Anywhere, London SE9 TNR. Tel: 020 8841 4712

It is not particularly valid for you, as the therapist, to make a judgement on the success or failure of your therapy with a client. The important marker is *how the client sees it*. This is what will really tell you what you have achieved. In simple terms, the mere fact of clients returning for further therapy sessions gives you a hint, and should be noted.

There are a variety of reasons why clients terminate therapy that have nothing to do with its quality, such as a simple problem simply solved, a change in external circumstances that made life look brighter, financial restraints, etc. However, if too many clients stop after one session you should look for an explanation. This issue would usually be discussed during supervision.

The role of experience

It is probable, when you set up in independent practice, that you will regard building up a client base as the initial goal. This means it is likely you will wish to offer your services to a wide clientele, with a variety of problems. If you are to be truly helpful, and not endanger your clients, this brings into question of your previous practical experience. While the majority of training courses stipulate a minimum number of practical counselling hours that you must complete in order to gain your diploma, some are quite non-specific as to what type of counselling you should be undertaking. We have come across trainees working, for example, as 'volunteers' in hospitals with little supervision except from a line manager, which a counselling course accepted as valid 'experience'. (It is possible, of course, that it may have been, but, equally, it may not.)

Think carefully about what experience you have to offer. Do you specialise in a particular area – e.g. bereavement, young people, victims of crime, substance abuse? Do you wish to continue as a specialist in one of these areas? Where you wish to broaden your clientele, and to deal with new, and perhaps difficult, problems, our advice is fourfold:

1   Be honest with yourself about your capabilities, and do refer onwards if need be. Against this, do not be too hard on yourself: the skills you have learned in other environments may well equip you to deal with new difficulties.
2   Book extra supervision and/or personal therapy to help you when dealing with new client problems. This self-development will not only give you extra confidence, but also practical guidance on best practice.
3   Read, read, read! We would encourage you to develop the most comprehensive home library that you can afford – perhaps make one of your development goals to purchase at least one new book per month. Subscribe to book lists from publishers such as Routledge and ensure that, whatever problems the clients bring you, if your knowledge of that particular area is limited, it certainly is not by the next time you see them! Even if you lose, or refer on, a client you feel too inexperienced to deal with on this occasion, make this a positive learning experience, take it to supervision, read and learn as much as you can, so that you will be well prepared on the next occasion.
4   Watch out for short courses and workshops on client difficulties that often come up for you. They are usually a very good investment. Your professional association will regularly send you details of these. Again, build these into your self-development, but focus specifically on areas of weakness.

A constant debate continues regarding the amount of weight that experience carries for a successful therapy outcome. So have confidence in yourself and if you consistently learn and develop, your practice will grow with you.

The European dimension

While the European dimension may be the last topic on your mind, do be aware that some British therapists may currently work in any European country. However, this could change in the future as, in other countries in Europe, the forms of training in the UK are not given the same recognition as the training undertaken by psychologists, and it is psychologists or psychiatrists who undertake most counselling and psychotherapy work in these countries.

The consequences could be twofold. First, if you at any point wish to work on the continent (or even relocate there for work or family reasons), you will need to ensure you are up to date with any work restrictions. Second, it is also possible in the future that, even working in the UK, therapists will be asked to submit to standardised rights to practise with the rest of Europe. The European Association of Psychotherapy can be contacted for further information. Their address is PO Box 6699, Dublin 2, Ireland. At the European level, appropriately qualified psycho-therapists can apply for the European Certificate in Psychotherapy through the European Association for Psychotherapy (see www.europsyche.org).

Additionally and from a positive perspective, we may be able to exchange ideas and ways of working, learning from alternative approaches that we have perhaps been less familiar with.

Reflection issues
- Do you believe that you have the right training and experience to move into private practice and, if not, what additional training/experience do you need?
- How are you going to evaluate the service you offer?
- Are you interested in the European dimension?

PROFESSIONAL BODIES

Why join a professional body?

For most therapists, joining a professional body is an obvious objective. However, some therapists wonder about the value of joining. Comments from counselling trainees include 'Sounds good on my CV', 'My agency requires it' and so on. As we progress through training and work experience, we become more aware of the value of joining a professional body, and also, that we have options as to which one to join.

Most (but not all) professional bodies connected to counselling offer a variety of different membership levels. The two most commonly applied for are:

• Membership of the professional body.
• Accreditation by that organisation (discussed further in the next section).

The main advantages of becoming a member of a professional association, especially for those in private practice, are:

• It sets a standard of professionalism for your practice that will be welcomed by at least your more discerning clients.
• Through its journals, it offers you the constant opportunity to keep in touch with the counselling world, the viewpoints of others, new information regarding practice ethics and essentials, books, courses and research findings.
• Professional organisations have a code of ethics and practice that their members must abide by. This code of ethics actually offers the practitioner a series of guidelines for good practice while adding to the therapist's credibility with clients.
• Information lines at the organisation's headquarters will usually be able to help with the multitude of miscellaneous queries that crop up for therapists, from 'Where can I find good insurance cover?' to 'How do I start the accreditation process?'
• For your client, such membership offers the safety of a complaints procedure, should a client feel that the therapy has been damaging to them in any way.
• Most professional therapeutic bodies hold a public Register of Members which enables potential clients to learn about your services.

Accreditation

While membership of a professional body is a helpful start, in itself it offers no yardstick as to the standard of work of the therapist. Most organisations are happy to take anyone who can show that they are involved in therapy in some way or another, as a Member, Student Member, Associate Member, or whatever. Being an Accredited, or Registered, Member is a different issue altogether, and it requires a different process to achieve this status. The accreditation process, while providing a benchmark for good practice and thus assisting the client in their search for a therapist, is also one that takes time, effort and energy, which many therapists may find it hard to make allowance for.

This may make accreditation sound onerous to those of you who have yet to make this leap, and there is an element of truth in this. For the accreditation process to be too easy would defeat the purpose, which is to test, against a set of consistent criteria, a therapist's ability to practise safely and ethically. In addition, there are those who question whether accreditation makes any real difference to client protection at all.

However, responsible and experienced practitioners will have little concern about their ability to successfully complete the process. It requires time, thought and an ability to demonstrate theoretical training, practical experience and personal counselling philosophy in a variety of ways. There is also a great deal of help and direction available, through comprehensive instructions issued with the accreditation forms and via counselling 'consultants' available to assist you on a one-to-one basis if you need it. A number of books and short (usually one-day) courses dedicated to the accreditation process and how to get through it are also of help.

We have, however, met a number of experienced, professional therapists who have not taken up accreditation to a professional body, and they have offered sound reasons for this. One reason for not becoming accredited is the cost; another is a concern about its value.

At present, while counselling is not statutorily regulated, registration/ accreditation provides the only standard by which ongoing competence to practise can be measured. Should you wish to offer your services to other organisations or the corporate market, such a professionally recognised standard could make a difference as to whether you get the work or not. For a long time one of the authors was the only accredited therapist in her area and it became evident that one of the reasons her practice was doing so well was because both referral sources and clients chose her in part because of her accredited status. Although being accredited does not automatically mean a therapist is better than a non-accredited one, this was not the view of those making contact.

For a self-employed therapist, competing with other therapists for clients, any edge is helpful. As more therapists become accredited, rightly or wrongly it can make it harder for those who are not. As the public becomes aware of accreditation and sees the bulk of therapists advertising this fact, they may well think that those who are not accredited are either inexperienced or not as good as those who are. We are sure that stating this view will cause some disquiet. However, it is given from a purely pragmatic point of view regarding securing clients, which, after all, is what a self-employed therapist has to do to survive.

Some practitioners are undecided as to which is the best professional association to become accredited by. There is quite a variety of organisations, depending on your counselling orientation or philosophy. One way of deciding is to consider which organisation is best known. Your path forward will be more straightforward if your accreditation is easily recognised and understood, rather than obscure and little known.

It is worth noting the Health Professions Council may eventually have a formal registration system for counsellors, psychotherapists and other caring and health professionals.

Reflection issues
- What are your views about joining a professional body?
- Which professional bodies are you eligible to join?
- If you are not already accredited or registered, would you consider this and why?

PROFESSIONAL ADMINISTRATION

Note-taking

Note-taking – keeping a written record of your therapy sessions with clients – has always been regarded as very much 'up to the therapist'. Some counselling agencies have standard procedures, but even within the lines and boxes that therapists must fill in there is a great deal of subjectivity as to what, and how much, is entered.

At one end of the scale, some therapists do not keep written notes at all. This is for a variety of reasons, ranging from forgetting, not having enough time, not being bothered, or concern over legal requests for the notes, to a personal view that it somehow interferes with the process of the therapy.

Our own view is that not keeping notes is unprofessional and a cause for concern. Imagine a doctor who did not keep notes and relied totally on memory to keep your medical history in his or her mind. Imagine a case where you found yourself in court, with a barrister raising an eyebrow at you and saying, 'So you are telling the court that you can't remember the exact content of your counselling sessions with Miss X over the last two years?'

We will assume that you are a therapist who is willing to keep notes, and may wonder at the best format for them. This will be decided by the question, 'What is the purpose (or purposes) of keeping client records?'

The most basic details – name, address and telephone number – are vital in case you need to change your meeting time at short notice. This information is contained on the Client Details Form, but in addition to this you might also want to keep your clients' telephone numbers with you, perhaps by using a code in your diary or personal organiser. After all, you could find yourself on a platform following an unexpected series of train cancellations with a client due to attend.

Apart from acting as an *aide-mémoire*, note-taking allows the therapist to record considered views about what has happened in the session. However, all therapists need to be aware that it is not in their best interests to record process comments, as these could prove detrimental to either the therapist or the client in a court of law. As with other professions, the move is more towards recording factual information only.

As your caseload builds, you will find it more difficult to recall the individual problems of each client, and the stage in therapy that you have reached with them.

Meanwhile, each client will be extremely mindful of exactly where they are at, and will not appreciate your not being at exactly that point with them.

Some clients who end therapy may return at a later stage and it is obviously helpful if you can easily remind yourself of previous work you did with these clients. Some counsellors feel that this is not an important issue, as they believe that when a client returns after a break it is rather like starting again with a new client, as the person will have moved on.

Taking client notes to supervision makes it much easier to work specifically with individual client problems – and also to check, when the supervisor makes a suggestion, whether you have already attempted this, and what the outcome was.

As has already been mentioned in this text, you may at some point be legally required to submit either your notes, or a report on your notes, to a court of law. We would suggest that whatever style of note-keeping you choose to follow, you ensure it is consistent. Your notes will, ideally, record all the practical information on the client that you need.

Once you have collected all the practical information that you need in your notes, you will begin to write your assessment of the client's problems, both as they present them to you, and any further, underlying problems you consider that they have. You may also wish to make notes about the client themselves – their demeanour, their non-verbal behaviour, and visual indicators (i.e. how they present themselves) that give you more clues about them. However, the more information of this nature that you make a note of, the more subjective you become and, as stated earlier, this can leave you and or/the client vulnerable should your notes be called upon.

A good question to ask yourself is, 'If I needed to write a report, précising the work that I have done with this client, would I be able to write one that was clear and factual, and included what was important?'

To review the legal position on client notes, refer back to the section of the book on legal requirements (see pp. 67–82).

Supporting documentation (e.g. Client Information Sheet)

Besides your note-taking, you will very often build up a file of miscellaneous documents for each client, which you will also need to keep carefully, safely and confidentially. You may, for example, wish to keep a separate client sheet recording such things as the person's basic details, start date, session times, any medication, GP details, and their session payments – how they paid, whether there are any fees outstanding, whether they have been invoiced, whether you have given them a receipt.

You may receive letters from, or write letters to, your client. You may write, on your client's behalf and with their permission, to third parties. You may ask your clients to fill in assessment questionnaires or keep treatment plans for them. They may give you copies of work they have done outside the session, or other documentation that they would like you to see. In this regard, we would recommend the early purchase of a small desktop photocopier, as soon as your practice can afford it.

Written communications (e.g. how to write a referral letter)

While accepting the principle of client confidentiality as paramount, there may be occasions when you will, with your client's permission, wish to write to a third party about your client: for example, when you are referring your client on for treatment, or when you are liaising with his or her GP or psychiatrist.

In writing such a letter, the issue of achieving a balance between being overly wordy and giving too little information to be helpful may cause uncertainty.

The main framework for such letters is usually as follows:

- Client background including how they were referred to you and the presenting problem.
- What the client's current difficulties are.
- Any medication that the client is on (relevant to their problems).
- Other treatments they may be receiving, or specialists they are seeing.
- Psychotherapeutic treatment suggestions (or treatment updates).

This information will be tailored, depending on whom the letter is being sent to, and it is wise to keep in mind the question, 'What would I need to know in order to best help this person?'

In addition, to ensure transparent communication, even though you have asked the client's permission to write to the person concerned, it would be helpful to the therapeutic process to provide the client with a copy of any such letter. You may also wish to consider whether you want your client to sign a simple permission slip clearly stating that they give their full permission for you to contact the person in question.

It is possible that some excellent therapists may worry that they are not very good letter writers. Write simply and clearly and ensure that you include all the important points. This will be more appreciated than an elaborate effort that may lack clarity.

Reflection issues
- Do you think it is unprofessional not to maintain records or notes of your therapy sessions?
- What note-keeping structure do you currently use and does it need amending in any way?
- Do you have a system for dealing with aspects such as client documentation etc.?

SUPERVISION

The special needs of those in private practice

BACP accredited therapists are expected to have a minimum of one-and-a-half hours of personal supervision per month for those months when they are seeing clients. Therapists who are not accredited would be wise to use this as a yardstick for their own supervision. Of course many therapists have more than one-and-a-half hours of supervision a month, depending on their caseload and any particular challenges these cases may bring.

There are special arguments for the use of supervision for therapists in private practice. Private practice is, in a sense, an isolated occupation. It is unlike working within a counselling agency or organisation, where you usually have constant opportunities for dialogue, peer supervision, theoretical discussions and an awareness of the practice methods of others. You may have one-to-one and/or group supervision provided by the service, whereas working alone means that, where you wish to provide yourself with such opportunities, you need to be pro-active in arranging both formal and informal supervision.

Types of supervision

There is a variety of different supervision options. Initially, let us consider what we actually expect to take to, and bring from, supervision. While we have found numerous texts which describe, in overview, the purpose of supervision, it is less easy to find descriptions of what therapists might expect from an individual session, and how they might evaluate its benefit other than via a 'feel good' (or 'feel bad') factor.

We have also discovered, in conversation with therapists, that many of them have no real idea of the ideal framework for a supervision session, and tend to 'muddle along', bringing with them whatever springs to mind at the time. For this reason, we would suggest that, as well as counselling texts, the independent practitioner reads some of the excellent texts on supervision, and what to expect from it. Reading in this area is often neglected by therapists, but can be hugely helpful for maximising the benefits of an integral part of your practice.

You may well place reliance on your supervisor to provide the framework for each session and for the ongoing development of your supervision. However, how will you know whether you are getting the best support that you can, without a good idea yourself of what this constitutes? Taking responsibility for self-evaluation can help you to answer this question. Constantly review whether the work you have done in supervision has led to a better understanding of any problems you have and whether it has enabled you to make better progress with difficult clients; whether it is assisting you to provide answers to tricky questions (e.g. onward referrals or legal dilemmas); and whether you feel you are developing competency as a therapist through it. Perhaps you feel too comfortable and seldom challenged during your supervision sessions. If this is the case, are you sure that you, and ultimately your clients, are benefiting from your supervision?

You may find that you gain greatest benefit from mixing supervision styles. For example, you may have one key supervisor but also join a peer group or have another supervisor who has more experience in an area that your current supervisor does not. In addition, you could opt for a more formalised group supervision arrangement and team up with a colleague for a peer supervision arrangement. The type(s) of supervision you decide upon are likely to be influenced by the work that you do, your experience and the pressures of your caseload.

Reflection issues
- How effectively do you feel you use your supervision time?
- Are you too comfortable and seldom challenged during your supervision sessions?
- What changes would you need to make, if any, if you were in private practice?

NETWORKING

How and why?

For a therapist in private practice, there is a variety of reasons why networking is important. These include:

- Getting yourself known to others, which may lead to referrals.
- Keeping up to date theoretically by attending courses, and engaging in dialogue with other health professionals.
- Keeping in touch with other like-minded professionals.
- The opportunity to offer help yourself to others where you have specific experience of, or information about, a problem they are dealing with.
- The opportunity to observe other therapeutic environments.
- Enabling yourself to keep a broad view of the profession, and what is going on within it.

Networking opportunities tend to fall into obvious areas – talking to colleagues, friends and associates, attending courses, conferences and workshops (or running them yourself) and joining relevant associations. Where you are using networking to increase your client base, consider where referrals are likely to come from – GPs? Solicitors? Local groups? Make an effort to contact them or attend events that they may frequent.

As mentioned in Part One, it is advisable to have a business card and networking is where your card comes into its own.

How many times have you come across a possible lead or contact, only to find that you are desperately searching for a pen and the back of an envelope in order to let them have your important personal details? Not only does this sometimes end in failure, but, at the very best, it looks totally unprofessional.

A good first step in designing your card is to collect a few from other people and see which you like best. Then think about your personal preferences:

- Would you like some sort of logo or graphic on it, or do you prefer a more conservative (possibly, more professional) approach?
- Are you happy about having personal details on your card such as your address, e-mail, etc.? Would you feel more comfortable giving your phone number only?
- What about your qualifications? Do you consider this a bit 'over the top' or essential if you wish to appear professional and genuine?

One point that often taxes people is whether to include 'counsellor', 'psychologist', 'psychotherapist' or whatever your preferred description of your professional status is. Putting it on the card certainly makes your role clearer, especially if it is months before the person you give it to looks at it again, or they pass it on to someone else.

It is a good idea to make a plan for networking, rather than to leave things to chance and an 'If something turns up I will go along' approach. Networking takes time and energy, but you would do well to regard it as an important part of building up your practice. Make a One-Year Network Planner (just a simple sheet of paper will do). Divide your planner into months, filling in details of courses and events you plan to attend, and then see where the gaps lie. Work out how much time you feel you can give to this activity on a monthly basis.

Attempt to balance the weeks and months so that your networking is ongoing, but not taking up too much of your time in any one period. Attempt to vary the type of networking that you do between the varieties of possibilities we have referred to above, and be pro-active in looking at new ideas. As you become more confident, both as a therapist and as a networker, you might consider offering to give a lecture or presentation. There is usually a variety of local groups and organisations looking for someone who can give an interesting talk to its members on almost anything. It may be therapy in general, or a talk on a specialist topic such as reducing social anxiety or increasing self-esteem.

Reflection issues
- What do you want to put on your business card?
- What networking activities do you currently engage in?
- If you were operating a private practice, what networking activities would you need to develop?

MEDICAL/PSYCHIATRIC BACK-UP

At some point in your career, it is likely that you will come across a client, or clients, whose problems you consider too severe for you to deal with yourself. In such cases, the option of onward referral can provide a solution, both for you and for the client needing help. How you come to such a decision will be based on a variety of factors, as described below. What is important is to have a policy and the relevant procedures in place, so that if and when this happens you can deal with it professionally and competently.

Where you become concerned about a client, we suggest that your first contact should be with your supervisor.

Knowing where to refer a client on to

It is a good idea to have on file a list of specialist agencies for problems you are not experienced in, or do not wish to deal with. These agencies should include those who can help with alcohol problems, drug problems, psychosexual difficulties, physical abuse, issues for children and young people, homelessness, etc. Having this information can also be useful if it comes up in therapy that someone close to the client needs help, and your ability to offer a source of help and advice will be much appreciated, as well as extremely helpful to the person concerned.

Before you make a decision as to a client's psychological problems, never rule out physical problems. If you are stumped by a client's description of his or her symptoms, always suggest a medical check-up. Do not assume that the pains in your client's arms or his shaking hands are due to anxiety, no matter who has assessed this as the case.

As an example, one of the authors was asked to see a client by a doctor, who had diagnosed acute anxiety in his patient. She presented with physical symptoms quite appropriate to this diagnosis – shaking and trembling, and dizziness that seemed to accompany every anxious thought that she had.

However, during her initial assessment it came to light that this client drank an average of nineteen cups of coffee a day. No wonder she was trembling and shaking! This was one issue that it had not occurred to her to ask her GP about. When she was referred back to the GP, he helped her wean herself off her caffeine addiction and she fully recovered.

There are the clients who may present, either initially or gradually, as therapy progresses, as having the type of severe psychiatric problem that it would be beyond your remit to deal with. If this happens, do not feel either pressured or inadequate. You simply need to be able to recognise mental illness of a type that needs medical help and know where, and to whom, to turn, to ensure that the client is placed in safe hands.

If it is possible for you to do so, a good idea when you set up practice is to make an appointment with your local doctors' surgery to be brought up to date with available NHS care for such clients. If the surgery has a Practice Manager, she may well be able to give you all the information you need. Discover how empathetic and knowledgeable the GPs are about mental health problems, whether they can offer psychiatric referrals (what the protocols are for this, likely waiting times, etc. are also useful questions to ask), and learn about the local Community Mental Health Trust.

Reflection issues
- Do you have an up-to-date referral list?
- What current systems do you use for medical/psychiatric back-up?
- What systems would you need to put into place if you were in private practice?

PERSONAL SECURITY

One of the questions we are asked by colleagues who work under an organisational umbrella is, 'Don't you feel frightened, having strangers come to see you when you are quite alone?' Let us consider your personal security position.

First, we are going to assume that when you work in your private practice, you are in an office at home where you are often on your own. So geographical location may be a first consideration. If your office is on the ground floor, and is very obviously a part of your home, the client may perceive it as linked to other rooms and there is no sense of isolation. Taking someone up to your attic might be a different issue.

Attempt to ensure that your counselling environment is light, bright and near to where other household members might be (even if there is no one there). One strategy you can use is that of leaving a radio or television on in a room that you pass by on the way to the therapy room (having ensured that it is not audible once you are in there). This leads the client to assume that there are other people at home, and gives you more confidence in your security.

Second, where do your clients come from? Restricting your clients to those who are referred from reliable sources may also minimise any difficulties. As a therapist in private practice, the reality is that there are clients that you might be skilled and happy to see in an agency or medical setting but that you would be unwise to see as a private practitioner. You have to think about the difference between the acceptance of 'some' inherent risk and an increase in risk factors.

Although we need to consider the possibility of attack we also need to recognise the rarity of such an event happening. However, it is still important to prepare ourselves, just in case. Obviously some counsellors may wish to help very disturbed or disordered clients. Private practice may not be the best environment for this type of work. However, let us just suppose that you are confronted by a client who seems to be becoming agitated in a way that suggests imminent violence. What precautions can you take, and what can you do?

- It is possible to have a 'panic button' installed in your office which is connected to your local police station. Of course, this may not be practical.
- Where do you sit in your office? If you sit nearer the exit door than your client, this will give you an advantage if you need to leave the room quickly. However, if the client can also have his or her way out of the office made easy, this may help him/her feel that they can escape too.
- Where you have the smallest doubt about a client in advance of a session, see if you can arrange for someone else to be around in the building (if all else fails, perhaps you could trade this with a neighbour for some babysitting time, for example). Better still, if you are really uncertain or uncomfortable about seeing this client, then perhaps you should seriously consider referring the client on.

With experience, most counsellors learn to detect the danger signals. Read books and papers on recognising the psychological manifestations of potential violence; attend courses on such issues if they are available. Signing on for self-defence training might give you a great deal of confidence, both in the consultation room and when walking home alone on a dark night, but it is always better to err on the side of caution. It is also important to remember that you need to keep your skills training fresh in your mind by attending refresher courses, otherwise you may well have forgotten what to do when you need to use it.

Finally, if you genuinely find yourself worrying about your personal safety in an office on your own, then it will probably affect the quality of your work and you may wish to think seriously about being in an independent practice on your own.

Alternatives could be to find other therapists who would be willing to share premises with you, or to respond to one of the various advertisements in professional journals with offers of rooms for hire along similar lines. Even renting a room in the local accountants' or solicitors' office is a possibility to consider. In the end, though this would be more costly, it might resolve your concerns over personal safety and allow you to work free from this worry.

CLIENT SECURITY

The suicidal client

Before you read further, we would like you to take a look at your counselling or therapy contract. Does it spell out, quite specifically, that counselling is completely confidential with the exception of any indication that the client may harm him- or herself or someone else? If it does not, we would suggest that you give very serious consideration to inserting this clause, or you may find yourself in an extremely difficult situation with a client who indicates that they are seriously suicidal.

Unless you take the view that a decision to end one's life is an ultimate expression of self-determination – in which case, keeping confidentiality would not be a problem – you will find yourself facing a dilemma. Even if this is your belief, the client's relatives may wish to take you to court for negligence if it were to surface that you realised suicide was a real risk and did nothing to intervene. Also, if you have not agreed with your client that where he presents a risk of self-harm this would need to be taken beyond the confidentiality of the therapeutic environment, and you do so, you could potentially open yourself up to being sued by the client.

For example, consider the consequences to the client of his doctor's role in having to provide reports on him for insurance or employment purposes. 'Attempted suicide' may not help his job prospects and he could even attempt to sue you for loss of earnings. So, before anything else, consider the legal position and check as to how well you have this covered.

This may also be a good time for you to consider (if you have not already done so) asking new clients for their GP details.

In practical terms, depending upon your client group, dealing with actively suicidal clients is not a daily experience, but you will need policies and procedures in place *ahead of time*, as, if the situation is acute, you may need to act very quickly.

The strength of your involvement with a suicidal client is going to depend very much on your own personal views and ethics. You may feel that therapeutic boundaries extend only so far as onward referral and securing client safety, or you may feel that you need to 'stay with' the client emotionally until they are, hopefully, stabilised.

Whatever action you decide to take, act as quickly as you can. You may decide, on speaking to the client, that making an emergency appointment in order to talk issues through with them may be adequate while you assess the situation. Announcing suicidal intentions, rather than simply carrying out the deed, does tend to imply a cry for help, so offering this initially may be both welcome and correct as a first response. However, if the need for help is not acknowledged, the client may well turn intent into action.

From this point onwards, you still need to make the decision regarding onward referral. The client themselves may be of help to you here, as they may also wish to be offered further treatment and medication. In any event, where you consider the suicidal threat to be serious, even if you believe it is now contained and minimised, we would advise you to write to (or telephone, of course, in an emergency) the client's GP. This does give you some element of shared responsibility for the client.

While we may be stating the obvious, do make fairly detailed notes of exactly what has happened, the sequence of events and the response of medical services, as soon as possible. This information will be required if for any reason the matter is taken further and you need to provide evidence or a written report.

It is never possible to be entirely sure of the circumstances in which you may meet such a problem or of your reaction to facing this situation for the first time. However, having your own guidelines in place ahead of time will do much to ensure that you deal with issues as professionally as possible and feel at least moderately comfortable with your actions.

In addition, when you are in private practice you need to consider how you would handle a situation where, for example, a suicidal client is the last client you see, at 8 p.m. in the evening. You have serious concerns, so what should you do? In situations like this there are no foolproof plans. However, it would be helpful to know, for example, that accident and emergency units have an on-call duty psychiatrist or that it is possible to arrange for a domiciliary visit by a mental health practitioner.

PART THREE

Personal self-management skills

In Part Three we focus on your personal self-management skills and ask you to reflect on some of the remaining issues not mentioned previously. This is an interactive section which may require a pen or pencil to tick items and note down your strategies for dealing with potential problems and stressors.

If you are already in private practice you may wish to skip the next couple of pages, although it may still be beneficial to recall what influenced you to take this path.

WHY DO I WANT TO RUN A PRIVATE PRACTICE?

Whereas many of your colleagues may appear to be quite happy working as counsellors or psychotherapists within a counselling centre, NHS general practice, college or university context, why did you one day decide, 'I want to set up in private practice'? Perhaps it is worth reflecting on this important career life change that has the potential to bring excitement, hard work and challenge. For some counsellors it also triggers anxiety.

Look at the checklist below. Tick the items that have encouraged you to consider going into private practice.

- Desire for independence
- Additional income
- Boredom or being fed up with current position
- Strong dislike of the restrictions of my current post
- Desire for more flexible working hours
- Wanting new challenges

- Ambition
- Liking taking risks
- Being upset by conflicts with other personnel in current post
- Lack of facilities in current post
- Feeling oppressed by the current regime or system
- Being fed up with the office politics of the current job
- Preferring my own company
- Wanting to have a sense of achievement
- Now fully qualified and going into private practice is a career progression
- Wanting to stand on my own two feet
- Desiring to work from home due to family commitments or other reasons
- Interest in supervising other counsellors
- Wanting to see a wider variety of clients and range of issues compared to existing situation
- Other reasons:

_____

_____

_____

_____

These are just a few of the reasons our colleagues and supervisees have given us for going into private practice. You may have included additional reasons too. Before we progress any further, please return to the checklist and reflect on the items you ticked. Ask yourself the following questions:

- Is this a good enough reason to go into private practice?
- If I shared these reasons with my colleagues and friends, would they agree?

Overall, is the balance of answers weighing in favour of going into private practice? If you are working systematically through this book, you now have a reasonable idea of what is involved.

Perhaps it would be advisable to note down the pros and cons of going into private practice. In the following example, Jayne completed her Making Choices Form to help her decide whether or not to take the plunge. Note how often the pros can also have cons! Please complete the blank Making Choices Form inserting the relevant issues that you noted earlier in this section. You may wish to enlarge this form on a photocopier, copy the form by hand onto A4 paper or produce a similar form on your PC. This evaluation of the advantages and disadvantages is personal to you, although you may share some of those Jayne encountered. If there are cons, attempt to take control by noting down how you might deal with them.

MAKING CHOICES FORM

> ### State problem or issue: *Going into private practice*

PROS	CONS
Total independence from any organisation.	*This could be scary!! However, this is my second job change in my life. I've survived it before.*
I can work from home and at the time I choose to.	*I may see some clients when my partner is out at work. This could be a risk. Need to consider this issue.*
I'll be able to see my children more easily.	*Working from home may mean that it will intrude into my personal life. At the moment, I leave work at the office.*
After about one year of private practice I may earn more than I do now.	*Financially it could be touch and go for the first six months. However, I do have some savings which I could fall back on if necessary.*
I'll avoid all the petty arguments at work.	*I could have learnt how to ignore them. At least it was a good distraction.*
I need a change as I'm becoming bored. I'll start looking forward to work again.	*Work may be a bit boring but at least I know what I'm doing. I always have my colleagues for support. I'll need to ensure I have frequent and adequate super-vision when in private practice.*
I can choose how many clients I can see in a day.	*I will need to learn more self-discipline. No more taking time off work for colds as I won't earn enough!*
	I'll be responsible for my accounts. However, I will be guided by my accountant.

© Centre for Coaching, 2003

MAKING CHOICES FORM

State problem or issue:

PROS	CONS

Now you have completed this exercise we hope you are still keen to go into private practice. If not, perhaps you may wish to consider other strategies to deal with potential disadvantages.

This small but important section has probably taken up to an hour to complete. Although it might have been very useful to have undertaken the exercise in Part One, until you had considered all the different issues that were raised in both Parts One and Two, you may not have been aware of what was involved. It is always difficult to know what we do not know. In this book, we wanted to take some of the chance or luck out of the equation.

DO I HAVE ENOUGH STAMINA?

How might you cope under pressure with hard work, low income, little support, working on your own? You may feel tired just thinking about this! Stamina is a quality that is behavioural, physical and psychological. Of course, when you are setting up a private practice, everything may go well. Successful action leads to motivation which stimulates the mind and energises the body. However, when you are having to work hard and not necessarily achieving high income or positive feedback from non-existent colleagues, and with few clients, stamina may be hard to muster. The implication here is that underpinning stamina is an attitude of mind that focuses on the goal and does not become distracted by occasional adversity or problems. In fact, this is good news since it means that most people can improve their stamina and motivation if they focus on modifying what they are telling themselves.

THE STRESSES OF PRIVATE PRACTICE

Although psychotherapists have a long history of private practice, the first recorded instance of a counsellor in private practice in Britain was in 1956 (Syme, 1994). In the past fifty years the figure has risen to thousands. Yet, many of us have experienced problems that are inherent to private practice. So what are the specific stresses that you are likely to encounter that need to be addressed?

- Economic stress, e.g. irregular income, especially while becoming established, cash flow problems, no income during holiday breaks.
- More physically tiring in later years.
- Environmental stress if practising from home, e.g. noise, unexpected visitors, no receptionist, no dedicated room for counselling.
- Environmental stress if practising in a health centre and renting a room, e.g. room used by others, external noise, unsuitable furniture and decoration.
- Competition from other practitioners.
- Unsociable hours, e.g. evening work.
- Working in isolation.
- No cover when ill.
- Lack of administrative support.
- Clash of values, e.g. charging clients.

Which stressors did you recognise? Reflect for a few minutes on how you can attempt to deal with them. Note down your answers below:

_____

_____

_____

_____

_____

_____

_____

Were there any easy answers? If not, you may find it helpful to discuss them with an experienced colleague, especially a therapist who is already in private practice. If you are not convinced that these potential stressors are worth dealing with, let's just consider a few of them.

The economic worries and concerns can be debilitating if a therapist allows them to become an overwhelming issue. Although a good business plan helps, often it is the negative 'fortune-telling' a person uses that is the real problem: 'It's going to turn out bad. I'll never have enough clients to survive.' Thinking errors such as fortune-telling may trigger anxiety before an event has even happened. We will return to thinking errors and how to deal with them later, as they are responsible for so much stress.

If you are intending to practise within a health centre and hire a room for a set time and day, it is likely that you will have a receptionist and possibly some administrative support. You may also have a steady stream of clients. The downside can be that you may not have been directly responsible for the furniture, room layout and so on. This can be tiresome, especially if you have to share the room with other practitioners who rearrange it whenever they practise. Although you may need to compromise, on certain issues, such as soundproofing the room, as a therapist, you will not be able to accept reduced standards.

To keep overheads down and for convenience, you may have decided to set up your practice at home, which leads to its own inherent problems. You will have considered these issues in your business plan but not necessarily the impact upon you directly. It can be even more difficult if you live with children, with unexpected noise or intrusions. It is important to consider the pros and cons of a home practice very carefully. In addition, there may be problems relating to your personal security and safety if practising from home alone. Of course, personal safety can be an issue in all locations. This was discussed in Part Two (see page 56). A personal safety risk assessment should be undertaken on a regular basis.

ARE YOU WORKING AT YOUR OPTIMUM OR EXPERIENCING BURNOUT OR RUSTOUT?

It has been suggested that, as we age, we may find tasks more tiring. Although our metabolic rates may gradually slow down, often feeling tired may be more a state of mind than to do with age. However, pacing ourselves at any age is an important part of stress management. In private practice, some therapists may attempt to fit in many clients without leaving sufficient breaks between sessions or while neglecting to take adequate lunch breaks. This can be compounded by working unsocial and long hours with inadequate therapeutic supervision. On an occasional basis, working long hours may be acceptable, but if this becomes the norm, then this could lead to stress, burnout and isolation. Figure 1 highlights the relationship between the ability to cope, pressure, rustout and burnout.

It is not just long hours that lead to burnout. Therapists who work in specialised areas such as rape, abuse or post-traumatic stress disorder may have many demands placed on them by their clients. Also, listening to these clients' negative life events and experiences can be stressful.

At the other end of the spectrum, counsellors who feel under-challenged may become bored and eventually experience rustout. If you recognise any of these issues, you may wish to consider what you can do about them. In some cases the options range from varying the workload or type of client problems dealt with, to changing jobs.

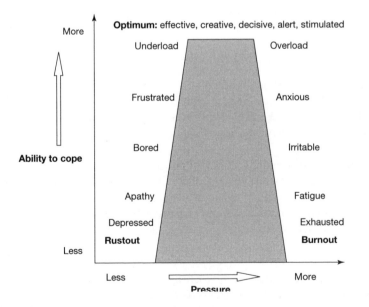

Figure 1
Source: Adapted from Palmer and Strickland, 1996

Where do you appear on the performance spectrum? On a day-to-day basis are you working at your optimum, being effective and creative, or fatigued or apathetic?

Reflection issues
- Why do you want to enter private practice?
- Have you ever felt isolated?
- How might you avoid either rustout or burnout?

COGNITIVE THINKING SKILLS FOR POSITIVE ACTION, MOTIVATION AND STRESS MANAGEMENT

As counsellors and psychotherapists we may look back to our childhood to see some of the causes or precursors of our problems as adults. Although this may be helpful in understanding ourselves, it does not always lead to changing our approach to work-related problems and stresses as they occur. In fact, our earlier experiences may have influenced how we view or perceive the world. However, even though we are not able to change what happened to us, we can use cognitive techniques to modify our perceptions and beliefs developed from the past about ourselves, work, colleagues and friends. These techniques are helpful in tackling procrastination, lack of motivation, stress and reduced performance. Potentially these are all important areas to deal with in private practice. In the next section we will focus on thinking errors.

Thinking errors and thinking skills

When we become stressed we usually have a variety of negative or unconstructive thoughts, which in turn prevent us from being able to resolve the problem effectively. Psychologists have identified fourteen common thinking errors. By identifying and challenging these thinking errors, we can reduce our stress levels.

As you read about the thinking errors below, ask yourself whether you have ever thought in this way, or whether one or more of these errors has ever prevented you from successfully resolving a problem or finding a solution. After each thinking error we suggest a thinking skill that may help to counter or challenge the error. We provide examples of the stress-inducing error and constructive stress-reducing alternative.

Labelling – error: negatively globally labelling yourself or other people instead of rating a person's skills or behaviours. For example, 'Because I've failed my counselling accreditation, I am a complete failure' or 'My colleague has made another mistake. This proves she is a total idiot and incompetent.'

De-labelling – skill: do you find labelling helpful in dealing with situations? Is this style of thinking motivating or de-motivating? Does it decrease or increase your anger? What happens to your stress levels? Does it make you feel happy?

Step back and ask how realistic and valid these global labels are. Are they an accurate description? Most people discover that it is less stressful to rate different aspects or deficits of ourselves or others instead of using a global rating. Constructive alternatives could be, 'Failing at my counselling accreditation does not mean I'm a complete failure as a human being' or 'When my colleague makes mistakes all it proves is that she is a fallible person like the rest of us.'

All-or-nothing thinking – error: viewing situations or problems only in extreme terms with no middle ground. For example, 'If I'm going to rent offices then I'll go for the best' or 'So many things are going wrong at work I may as well go into private practice.'

Relative thinking – skill: consists of attempting to find the middle ground or looking for shades of grey. Constructive alternatives could be, 'I don't have to go for the best, which is probably too expensive in the first year of private practice. Good enough will do' or 'Things may be going wrong at work but many things happen that are great or just okay too. Perhaps I should look at the overall picture and maintain a realistic perspective.'

Focusing on the negative – error: focusing on the negative aspects of a situation or event, while ignoring the positive. For example, when running a training workshop, dwelling on a few negative student feedback evaluation forms ('The course was boring'), rather than focusing on the overall comments; or ignoring any positive feedback given by your colleagues, 'They may think I've done a good job, but I made so many mistakes I really messed up that project.'

Focusing on the overall picture – skill: instead of just focusing on the negative, attempt to focus on the overall picture, including the positive. Constructive alternatives could be, 'Certain parts of the course were boring but there were good parts too' or 'In fact I made five mistakes and we reached the agreed targets.'

Discounting the positive – error: considering all positive events as unimportant and disregarding them. For example, 'I did well in the exam because the questions were easy', rather than acknowledging that you studied hard. Or, 'My manager only gave me a good appraisal because he doesn't want to upset me.'

Counting the positive – skill: when people do well or receive good feedback from others, they can choose to accept the positive results. Constructive alternatives could be, 'I did well in the exam because I worked hard on the course' or 'My manager gave me a good appraisal because I have made a big effort at work to achieve our goals.'

Magnification or 'awfulising' – error: exaggerating the significance of an event or problem out of all proportion. With stress it involves focusing on the negative, and is therefore sometimes known as 'awfulising'. For example, 'If I don't make sufficient profit in private practice it will be the end of the world' or 'It's absolutely awful not to pass my psychotherapy exams.'

Demagnification or 'de-awfulising' – skill: in most situations the outcome is seldom really awful or the end of the world, but our thinking makes it so. By making a mountain out of a molehill we lose sight of the whole picture. This is responsible for much unnecessary stress. Questions to counter this thinking include: What aspect of this situation is bad? Will it really be that important in three, six or twelve months from now? Is it really the end of the world? Am I losing sight of the overall picture?

Constructive alternatives could be, 'If I don't make sufficient profit in private practice I could always get paid employment again. This would be a pain but not the end of the world' or 'Failing my psychotherapy exams is a real hassle but hardly a horror. I can resit them.'

Minimisation – error: the opposite of magnification. It involves playing down the importance of our achievements and strengths. For example, 'Becoming a Registered Psychotherapist was nothing' or 'When I've done well, it's always down to luck.'

Taking personal responsibility – skill: consider what you are responsible for in a particular situation. Avoid downplaying your involvement. Take responsibility for your actions whether positive or negative. Constructive alternatives could be, 'At the time, I had to work hard especially when I was in training to become a psychotherapist' or 'On reflection, my good luck is in direct proportion to my hard work.'

Mind-reading – error: making assumptions that people are either thinking or reacting negatively towards us, based on a lack of evidence. For example, 'My colleague didn't acknowledge me in the corridor today, she must be angry with me' or 'My partner is unhappy with my business. She hasn't asked me about it for weeks.'

Considering possible alternatives – skill: stressed people have a tendency to interpret others' actions or behaviours in a negative manner. This is often based on little evidence. Challenge your mind reading. Consider the alternatives. Ask yourself: Are there any other possible reasons for the person's behaviour? Am I making a negative interpretation when I could make a positive interpretation? Constructive alternatives could be, 'Perhaps my colleague was deep in thought and didn't notice me' or 'Perhaps my partner is either preoccupied or believes that my business is going well.'

Fortune-telling – error: predicting a negative outcome for events despite the fact there is a lack of evidence to support this. For example, 'I'm bound to get into debt going into private practice' or 'The presentation will all go wrong.'

Reality check – skill: how realistic are your powers of negative clairvoyancy? Rate your predicted outcome of the particular event on a scale of 0 to 100, where 0 is certain not to happen and 100 is certain to happen. Constructive alternatives could be, 'If I carefully manage my private practice I am unlikely to get into debt' or 'I may make a few mistakes but it is unlikely that the whole presentation will go wrong.'

Personalisation and blame – errors: blaming ourselves for outcomes for which we are not entirely responsible. For example, 'My client's condition did not improve in spite of all my experience' or 'The team did not reach the targets and it's all my fault.' Blame is the opposite of personalisation. This is where you blame others, ignoring any personal responsibility your own attitudes or behaviours may have had for the outcome. For example, 'My clients do not improve as they are never willing to work hard' or 'Nobody told me that I had to pay VAT bills on time.'

Broadening the picture – skill: constructive alternatives to personalisation could be, 'I'm being unrealistic. I can't assume that all my clients will improve, regardless of my level of experience' or 'There's no "I" in team work. We were all equally responsible for the outcome.' Constructive alternatives to blame could be, 'I expected too much too soon from my clinically depressed clients' or 'I am responsible for finding out about VAT payments. In future I will take care to read the VAT forms.'

A useful technique to challenge personalisation or blame is to note down all the individuals or issues involved and then represent these different people and issues graphically on a pie chart. This will allow you to allocate everybody's responsibility for what happened, including yourself.

Case study (Palmer et al., 2003)

> *Situation*: Maureen was a manager of a large team. Maureen's department failed to reach their target and she felt totally responsible for the situation (personalisation) (see first pie chart). Maureen then used the 'broadening the picture' technique and realised she was not completely responsible (see second pie chart) and there were in fact other factors that had contributed to the team not meeting their target.

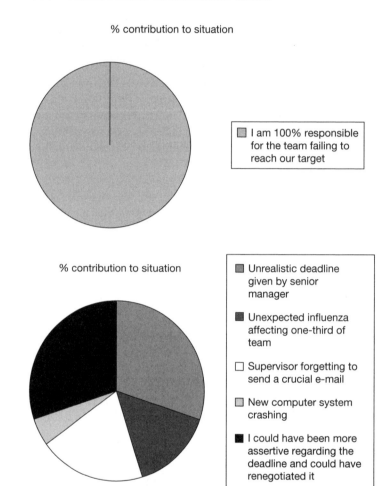

% contribution to situation

☐ I am 100% responsible for the team failing to reach our target

% contribution to situation

■ Unrealistic deadline given by senior manager

■ Unexpected influenza affecting one-third of team

☐ Supervisor forgetting to send a crucial e-mail

☐ New computer system crashing

■ I could have been more assertive regarding the deadline and could have renegotiated it

Case study (Palmer et al., 2003)

Situation: Robert's teenage son had just failed his exams. Robert completely blamed his son (blame) (see first pie chart). However, on reflection, once he had broadened the picture, he realised he was not completely to blame, and there were in fact other factors that had contributed to the situation (see second pie chart).

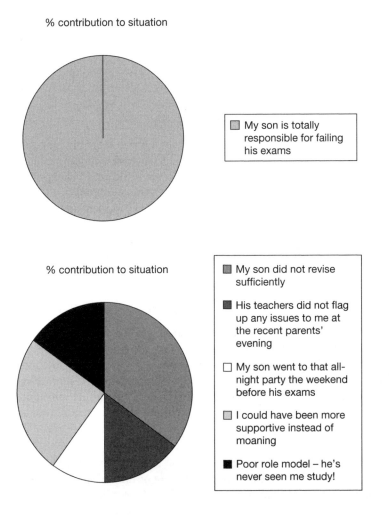

% contribution to situation

My son is totally responsible for failing his exams

% contribution to situation

My son did not revise sufficiently

His teachers did not flag up any issues to me at the recent parents' evening

My son went to that all-night party the weekend before his exams

I could have been more supportive instead of moaning

Poor role model – he's never seen me study!

Emotional reasoning – error: a situation is evaluated purely based on how you feel emotionally. For example, 'I feel like a complete idiot so I must be one', or 'I feel so anxious. Flying must be dangerous.'

Keeping emotions in their place – skill: remind yourself that just because you are feeling an intense negative emotion, it does not necessarily mean that you are in a stressful, anger- or anxiety-provoking situation. Check with your colleagues, friends or family whether the situation should provoke such an emotional response. Often people misunderstand a situation, they mishear what was said, misconstrue what was meant or do not have the facts. Constructive alternatives could be, 'Making mistakes does not mean I'm a complete idiot' or 'Although I may feel anxious, I need to remember the statistics that show flying is one of the safest forms of transport. In fact, I'm more likely to suffer a fatal accident in my home.'

Over-generalisation – error: based on one unfortunate event, drawing sweeping, generalised conclusions about all other events, usually with insufficient evidence. For example, 'That exam was so difficult, all the others will be too' or 'Because I didn't get that job, I'm unlikely to be offered any other post.'

Focus on the information available – skill: attempt not to draw inferences or conclusions based on little evidence. Wait until you have more evidence available before you draw conclusions. Constructive alternatives could be, 'Although that exam was difficult, I may find the others easier' or 'Not getting a job does not mean that there won't be other opportunities. I need to be persistent and carry on applying.'

'Demandingness' – error: this occurs when you hold fixed, rigid and absolutist beliefs often resulting in unrealistic expectations of yourself and others. These are usually expressed as 'musts', 'shoulds', 'got tos', 'have tos' and 'oughts'. For example, 'I must always arrive on time' or 'My staff must not make mistakes.'

Thinking more coolly and thinking flexibly – skill: challenge your demanding language. For example, 'Where is it written that I must?', 'Who said I should?', 'Is this flexible thinking?' Then introduce flexible, non-demanding, non-absolutist beliefs that consist of preferential wishes and desires. Constructive alternatives could be, 'Although it's strongly preferable to arrive on time, realistically sometimes I'll arrive late' or 'Just because I wish my staff did not make mistakes does not mean that they won't.'

'I can't stand it' – error: by telling yourself, 'I can't stand it' or 'I can't bear it', you reduce your tolerance to dealing with frustrating or difficult problems. For example, 'I can't stand my clients turning up late' or 'I can't bear doing boring paperwork.' This is known as low frustration tolerance (LFT).

Developing high frustration tolerance (HFT) – skill: acceptance of reality and the challenging of LFT beliefs are important. Ask yourself: 'Where is the evidence that I can't stand it?' 'How long have I been standing it?' The task, albeit quite hard, is to develop new beliefs that change LFT to HFT. Constructive alternatives could be, 'I may not like it but I'm living proof that I can stand clients turning up late' or 'If I just accept that sometimes I have to do boring paperwork, then I will be less frustrated and will complete it more quickly.'

Thinking errors audit

Before we go any further and include other thinking skills it would be an idea now to stop and take stock of the thinking errors you make on a daily basis or when you are in stressful situations. The exercise below will help you to focus on your thinking errors.

Thinking errors audit

Cooper and Palmer (2000) advocate undertaking a personal audit of thinking errors. Think about a past, current or future issue you are frustrated or stressed about. Write down your stress-inducing thoughts associated with the issue. Next, note the thinking errors you recognise in yourself.

Stress-inducing thoughts (SITs)

_____

_____

_____

Thinking errors	**Your example**
Labelling	
All-or-nothing thinking	
Focusing on the negative	
Discounting the positive	
Magnification	
Minimisation	
Mind-reading	

Fortune-telling

Personalisation

Blame

Emotional reasoning

Over-generalisation

'Demandingness'

'I can't stand it'

By identifying your thinking errors when you are stressed or under-performing, you will be in a better position to appraise the problem or pressures more realistically. This process of thinking about your thinking will help to distance you from your stress-inducing thoughts and the negative feelings that arise from them. Thus, even though this is an audit, it may help you to reduce stress and increase performance.

Additional thinking skills

In this section we cover a number of additional thinking skills which may help you to reduce stress and increase performance.

Befriend yourself: befriending is a powerful thinking skill that many of us already possess but seldom use on ourselves to counter unhelpful self-critical thoughts. When a colleague or friend makes an error, think about what supportive statements you generally make. It is likely that you are not critical or harsh. However, notice that you may be harsh on yourself in the same circumstances. So instead of thinking, 'I was useless at giving the presentation', stand back and think about it more realistically: 'Realistically in the whole hour I only made two or three errors. That's not bad considering it was my second presentation.' By accepting that you made errors but also by being supportive when you focus on the positive aspects, your internal dialogue will reduce stress and maintain motivation.

Look for evidence: challenge your stress-inducing ideas by looking for evidence, instead of making assumptions. Ask your friends, family or colleagues for feedback about a task you have undertaken, such as chairing a meeting, or giving a wedding speech. You can also test assumptions by deploying behavioural interventions: for example, if you believe 'I can't stand waiting for a train', make yourself arrive at the station earlier or wait for the next train. This will provide you with living proof that you are able to stand the waiting, even if you do not particularly like it. It is important to avoid mind-reading.

Questions to aid challenging your stress-inducing thinking and thinking errors

The use of challenging questions is an excellent method to help you examine the validity of your stress-inducing thinking and thinking errors. Think back to the earlier exercise when you noted down your thinking errors. Write down below your stress-inducing statement and thinking error. Then choose questions that help you to challenge its validity (Palmer and Strickland, 1996).

Stress-inducing statement or thinking error:

Is the belief logical?
- Would a scientist agree with it?
- Where is the belief written apart from in my own head?
- Am I labelling myself, or somebody or something else? Is this a logical thing to do?

Is the belief realistic (empirically correct)?
- Where is the evidence for my belief?
- Would people I know agree with my idea?
- Is the situation so awful or terrible? What is making it feel this way?
- Am I making a big deal of this? Am I blowing it out of proportion?
- If I 'can't stand it', what will really happen?

Is the belief helpful/pragmatic?
- Where is my attitude getting me?
- Is it helping me attain my goals?
- Is my belief helping me to solve my problem?
- Am I placing demands on others or myself? Is this helpful and constructive?
- Am I taking things too personally?

The questions listed below are designed to enable you to move forward to develop more effective beliefs (adapted from Palmer and Whybrow, 2004).

1   What are the consequences for my goals if I hold on to this belief?

2   Are there any advantages for me in holding on to this belief?
3   What is the evidence for and against this belief?
4   Would I teach this belief to my family/friends/colleagues?
5   What experiments could I conduct to test the truth or falsity of this belief?
6   In what way does this belief make sense to me?
7   If I was helping a friend, what suggestions would I make to someone with a belief similar to mine?
8   Do I still want to be stuck with this block in one/three/six months' time?
9   Is this belief rigid or flexible?
10   If I was giving advice to myself as an impartial observer, what suggestions would I offer to deal with this block?
11   If I was presenting my belief to a jury of my peers, is it likely they would be persuaded by my arguments?
12   How would I sum up the case for and against my belief?
13   What would be a more helpful belief to adopt in order to overcome this block?
14   How can I prove to myself that this belief is more helpful?

In the next section, when you are using the worksheets, these questions can be applied to help you to challenge your stress-inducing thoughts and performance-interfering thinking.

Stress Thought Record

Stress Thought Records involve noting down the thinking errors or the stress-inducing thoughts you are experiencing. These can be referred to as Stress Inducing Thinking (SIT). Once you have identified which thoughts are exacerbating your stress you can begin to apply the thinking skills discussed previously, and develop thoughts to alleviate the stress, known as Stress Alleviating Thinking (SAT) (developed by Neenan and Palmer, Centre for Stress Management).

Exercise

Below is an example of a Stress Thought Record. Complete the blank form for a problem you wish to feel less stressed about, or a fear you have about setting up your private practice. Note down in the SIT column any thoughts, attitudes or thinking errors you have that increase stress. Then use the questions and thinking skills from the previous sections to aid challenging your SIT and help you to develop SAT. Then complete the SAT column.

STRESS THOUGHT RECORD

Stress Inducing Thinking (SIT)	Stress Alleviating Thinking (SAT)
Redundancy could impact upon my family and finances	*Worrying won't decrease the likelihood of redundancy – it will probably make it worse if anything* *I have lots of skills. If I was made redundant I shouldn't have too much of a problem finding other employment*
This shouldn't happen to me	*Why shouldn't it? The reality is that cut-backs may have to be made*
The company should look after its staff	*The company has everyone to consider – it's not personal*
They are treating me so badly after all the years I've worked for them	*Are they? I'm taking this rather personally. It won't help me!* *Other ideas:* *When worry occurs at work, tell myself that, 'there's nothing I can do about it right now'* *Perhaps use worry time for a limited period in the evening* *Use problem-solving skills to work on employment situation and revise financial situation. Ask for break in mortgage payments* *Update CV. Scan papers for jobs*

Centre for Stress Management, 2001

STRESS THOUGHT RECORD

Stress Inducing Thinking (SIT)	Stress Alleviating Thinking (SAT)

© Centre for Stress Management, 2001

Improving performance under pressure

Do you wish to increase your performance when under pressure? Certainly when setting up and running your private practice you are likely to experience periods of high pressure and sometimes you may find that you are not achieving what you would like to. Or conversely when you are not under pressure you may find you waste time and become unproductive. In both of these circumstances it is possible that you may have Performance Interfering Thoughts (PITs). These can be noted down on the Enhancing Performance Form and new Performance Enhancing Thoughts (PETs) can be developed. This method was developed by Neenan and Palmer at the Centre for Coaching and is similar to using the Stress Thought Record. Below is a completed Enhancing Performance Form.

ENHANCING PERFORMANCE FORM

State problem: *Giving a poor presentation to a group of local health professionals*

Performance Interfering Thoughts (PITs)	Performance Enhancing Thoughts (PETs)
I 'MUST' perform well	*Although it's strongly preferable to perform well, realistically I don't have to*
Otherwise the outcome will be awful	*If I don't perform well, the outcome will be bad but hardly awful and devastating. Certainly not the end of the world!*
I'll never get that promotion	*All-or-nothing thinking and fortune-telling again! It's unlikely I'll be judged on one event*
This will prove I'm totally useless	*It may prove I have presentation skills deficits but not that I'm useless. Perhaps instead of avoiding presentations, in future I need to get more practice by offering to do them!*

© Centre for Coaching, 2003

ENHANCING PERFORMANCE FORM

State problem:

Performance Interfering Thoughts (PITs)	Performance Enhancing Thoughts (PETs)

Exercise

Think of a situation related to your work in which you wish to improve your performance. Note down in the PITs column any thoughts, attitudes or thinking errors you have that interfere with or reduce your performance. Then use the thinking skills or questions from the earlier sections as an aid to challenging your PITs. Then develop and note down in the PETs column your new Performance Enhancing Thoughts.

Imagery exercises

There is a range of imagery techniques that can help either to prepare us for potentially stressful or difficult situations that we may encounter or to motivate us (Palmer and Dryden, 1995). In this section we cover two important techniques, coping and motivation imagery – both may be necessary to help you set up in private practice.

Coping imagery

Coping imagery involves picturing yourself coping with the situation you are feeling stressed about and challenging the negative imagery that is winding you up. It is important to note that this is called 'coping imagery' not mastery imagery, whereby you imagine yourself completing the task perfectly (McMullin, 1986). Many people who are feeling stressed about a future feared event do not have the confidence to believe they will ever be able to 'master' the situation. However, they are able to imagine themselves coping because this allows for the realistic element of fallibility. For example, accepting you will be able to give a perfect conference paper is unlikely, but giving a paper that is good enough is more realistic.

Coping imagery can also help to deal with phobias or difficult social situations. It can also be useful to prevent negative images raising stress levels, which may later become self-fulfilling prophecies if not tackled.

Exercise

There are five steps in this exercise:

Step 1: Think of the future event you are feeling anxious or stressed about.
Step 2: Write down the particular aspects of this situation that you are feeling most stressed about.
Step 3: Think of ways to overcome these problems. You may want to speak with a friend or colleague if you are unable to think of a way to deal with the problem.
Step 4: Now visualise yourself in the situation that you fear, and, using the strategies you have identified in Step 3, slowly imagine yourself coping. Picture yourself dealing with the problems as they arise. You may need to repeat this procedure three or four times.

Step 5: Practise this technique regularly, especially when you find yourself feeling stressed about a situation or event.

Motivation imagery

Motivation imagery was developed by Palmer and Neenan (1998) to help demotivated people prepare themselves for action. It can be used for both personal and work-related problems. The first stage is to imagine not doing what you want to do for the rest of your life, and the second stage is to visualise actually doing what you want to do.

Exercise

Think about an area in your life that you could improve by taking action, which until now you have avoided. This could include setting up in private practice or leaving a relationship.

- Next visualise yourself for the rest of your life not undertaking the change. What effect will it have on you or your friends and family? What regrets would you have if you did nothing?
- Now, imagine yourself doing what you would like to do and think about the short- and long-term benefits that the change would make to your life.
- Finally, consider how you are going to put the change into action.

It is very important to visualise the 'inaction' imagery before the 'action' imagery, in order to motivate yourself. Do not use this technique if you are depressed.

Reflection issues
- Which thinking errors or beliefs could hold you back from progressing with your goal of setting up a private practice?
- Do you have any goal-blocking PITs? How could you tackle them?
- Would your clients find thinking skills useful?

TIME MANAGEMENT

Most newly self-employed people in any profession vastly under-estimate the number of non-chargeable hours they must work to support their chargeable hours. A number of newly self-employed therapists envisage clients entering and leaving during the day, accompanied by some client note-taking, after which they close the office door and move on to their social and domestic life. As the practice builds, other work offers are likely to appear.

If you are marketing your services, time will be required to keep on top of this – in addition to work preparation, letter writing, telephoning, face-to-face meetings, invoicing, note-taking, record-keeping, stationery ordering, trying to fix a recalcitrant computer, research, CPD courses, supervision (and, of course, the dreaded income tax return). Many practitioners operate on the 'wing and a prayer' principle that, if they work hard and conscientiously, somehow it will all fit together.

Perhaps you will choose to limit your client workload to a set number of individual client sessions per week – the 'keeping things simple' approach, which also keeps things fairly neat. However, if you wish to run a flourishing, full-time practice that includes lots of extra activities such as training, writing, corporate work, etc., you will need to learn to manage your time very effectively to avoid work overload and burnout.

Kate Hinch, a time management trainer, advocates six principles of good time management:

1   *Value your time*: Don't fritter it away on pointless tasks – it is a precious commodity that needs to be well spent if you are to succeed.
2   *Analyse and prioritise tasks*: Don't undertake tasks as they arrive on your desk, but think about their current importance in relation to other work you have to do.
3   *Know what to do – and what not to do*: Have a task list that incorporates your prioritised workload. If other things creep in, be firm with yourself about leaving them alone.
4   *Say 'no' when appropriate – and mean it*: One of the hardest things to do, especially with a new business, is to turn work away. You may want to accept every piece of work that comes your way, to build the business up and to earn money. You may believe that turning work away means that it will be the last work you are ever offered, and that you will live to regret saying 'no'. You must learn to do so, or you may find yourself so swamped that you are not working effectively, or on the work areas you find most challenging and productive.
5   *Spend time to save time*: In simple terms, doing things like spending a few minutes on note-taking immediately after the client has left becomes a priority.
6   *Don't procrastinate – do it now*: In other words, stop unbending those paperclips and gazing out of the window, and start making those difficult telephone calls to organisational clients whose payments are outstanding.

If time management is proving a problem, or if you want to pre-empt problems before they arise, you need to look closely at the amount of actual time you spend over, say, a week or a month on running your practice and the various tasks that involves. You need to discover the total number of hours these things take you to do.

Depending on the result of this, you may need to start to prioritise your activities and get rid of or minimise the less productive activities. We would suggest that the easiest way of achieving this is to keep a diary record over, say, a two-week period. You need to keep a record of your chargeable hours. When you have added all your activities together, divide your income by the total number of hours, and this is your true hourly rate.

There is a wide variety of time management models, and perhaps one of the most widely known is Steven Covey's 'Time Management Matrix' (1989).

Covey suggests dividing your 'To Do' list into four boxes:

1 Urgent and important
2 Important but not urgent
3 Urgent but not important
4 Neither important nor urgent

You will not have too much difficulty differentiating between what goes into each category. For example, under heading 1, 'Urgent and important', things such as the phone call you must make today to secure new business, the letter you need to write confirming a course attendance, the income tax return you need to have in the post by Friday – and so on. These activities are very necessary and driven by a 'here and now' urgency.

Covey suggests that the most important category to spend time on is number 2, 'Important but not urgent', as this is where all the real development goals lie. You will place under this heading reading, research, learning new skills, marketing your practice, reassessing your career goals, and anything else that will develop both yourself and your business, but which doesn't need to be done today.

Category 3, 'Urgent but not important', contains such tasks as paying a final demand for a newspaper bill or reaching the dry cleaners before they close.

Category 4, 'Neither important nor urgent', relates to things such as watching TV, unbending paperclips, social telephone calls, browsing around the shops, etc.

Unless you spend as much time as you can working with items under heading 2, 'Important but not urgent', it will be hard for your business to develop. While we tend to react to urgent matters, we take the initiative – we are more pro-active – with important matters.

Reflection issues
- How would you describe your time management skills?
- Which time management skills do you need to improve?
- If you procrastinate how could you choose to confront this behaviour?

RELAXATION

Thinking, imagery and time management skills are excellent strategies for stress management. However, many practitioners also find relaxation exercises very useful to help them deal with pressure and stress. Obviously, reading, walking or listening to music may help encourage a relaxed state of mind, but not for everybody. In this section we introduce three relaxation methods that have been found to be useful by many thousands of people to alleviate the physical effects of stress and tension. The techniques focus on switching off the sympathetic nervous system, which is the stress or arousal response, and stimulating the parasympathetic nervous system, which is responsible for relaxation and conserving your body's energy levels (Palmer *et al.*, 2003).

Do note that when undertaking the relaxation exercises described below you may experience odd sensations such as tingling or warmth in your hands or light-headedness. This is all part of the relaxation process. If you do not like these feelings simply open your eyes and they will quickly pass away.

Benson relaxation technique

The Benson Relaxation Response is a Western form of meditation that has been found to reduce hypertension and high blood pressure (Benson, 1976). It involves using a number of your choice, frequently the number one, as a mantra. Focusing on the number helps you to ignore any unwanted, negative or intrusive thoughts. With this technique there are a number of stages to follow.

Exercise

Stage 1: find a place where there is as little noise as possible, and you will not be disturbed.

Stage 2: either lie or sit in a comfortable position.

Stage 3: close your eyes.

Stage 4: relax your muscles in groups, starting with your face and moving down to your toes. This can be done by first tensing or squeezing a muscle, and then relaxing it.

Stage 5: focus on your breathing. Breathe in through your nose and out through your mouth. Avoid raising your shoulders as you breathe. Imagine you are breathing from your stomach, and notice how it may rise and fall as you breathe.

Stage 6: in your mind say a number every time you breathe out, such as the number 'one'.

Stage 7: continue doing this for 5–20 minutes.

Stage 8: finish in your own time. When you feel ready to stop, keep your eyes closed and sit or lie quietly for a few minutes.

If you find you are being distracted by other thoughts, let them pass and go back to repeating your chosen number. The important rule about relaxation is not to try too hard. With regular practice you will find that relaxation comes to you naturally, but it may take a while before this happens.

Relaxation imagery

Relaxation imagery can be a very effective way to relax body and mind. Palmer and Strickland (1996) suggest imagining yourself in your favourite relaxing place such as walking on a beach or sitting in a deck-chair in your garden. The exercise below highlights the method.

Exercise (Palmer and Strickland, 1996)

Step 1: find a place where there is as little noise as possible, and you will not be disturbed.
Step 2: either lie or sit in a comfortable position.
Step 3: close your eyes and picture your favourite relaxing place.
Step 4: concentrate on the colours in this place.
Step 5: concentrate on one particular colour.
Step 6: concentrate on the sounds in your place. It may be silence.
Step 7: imagine touching something in your place.
Step 8: concentrate on the aromas in your place.
Step 9: when you are ready, open your eyes.

By practising this technique on a regular basis, you will be able to achieve a relaxed state quickly and with minimal effort. It is also very helpful if you are experiencing sleeping difficulties or tension.

Multimodal relaxation technique

The Multimodal Relaxation Method was developed by Professor Stephen Palmer at the Centre for Stress Management to help clients attending therapy sessions and delegates attending stress management workshops to find the particular technique that suits them. It contains a number of different relaxation techniques including breathing, mantras, imagery, sounds, smell and touch (Palmer, 1993). Once you have tried the method, decide which technique you prefer for future use.

Below is the Multimodal Relaxation Method text, which you can either ask someone to read to you, or record yourself reading so that you can play it back later. Obviously, do not read out aloud the instructions to pause. (NB If you wear contact lenses either remove them before the exercise or do not look upwards.)

Begin by sitting comfortably on a chair and close your eyes. If at any time during the exercise you feel odd feelings such as tingling sensations, light-headedness, or whatever, this is quite normal. If you open your eyes then these feelings will go away. If you carry on with the exercise usually these feelings will disappear anyway.

If you would like to, listen to the noises outside the room first of all
Long pause
And now listen to the noises inside the room
Pause
You may be aware of yourself breathing
These noises will come and go throughout this session and you can choose to let them just drift over your mind or ignore them if you wish
Pause
Now keeping your eyelids closed and without moving your head, I would like you to look upwards, your eyes closed, just look upwards
Long pause
Notice the feeling of tiredness
Pause
And relaxation
Pause
In your eye muscles
Pause
Now let your eyes drop back down
Pause
Notice the tiredness and relaxation in those muscles of your eyes
Pause
Let the feeling now travel down your face to your jaw, just relax your jaw
Long pause
Now relax your tongue
Pause
Let the feeling of relaxation slowly travel up over your face to the top of your head
Pause
To the back of your head
Long pause
Then slowly down through your neck muscles
Pause
And down to your shoulders
Long pause
Now concentrate on relaxing your shoulders, just let them drop down
Pause
Now let that feeling of relaxation now in your shoulders slowly travel down your right arm, down through the muscles, down through your elbow, down through your wrist, to your hand, right down to your fingertips
Long pause
Let the feeling of relaxation now in your shoulders slowly travel down your left arm, down through your muscles, down through your elbow, through your wrist, down to your hand, right down to your fingertips

Long pause
And let that feeling of relaxation now in your shoulders slowly travel down your chest right down to your stomach
Pause
Just concentrate on your breathing
Pause
Notice that every time you breathe out you feel more
Pause
And more relaxed
Long pause
Let the feeling of relaxation travel down from your shoulders right down your back
Long pause
Right down your right leg, down through the muscles, through your knee, down through your ankle
Pause
To your foot, right down to your toes
Long pause
Let the feeling of relaxation now travel down your left leg
Pause
Down through the muscles, down through your knee, down through your ankle
Pause
To your foot, right down to your toes
Long pause
I'll give you a few moments now
Pause
To allow you to concentrate on any part of your body that you would like to relax further
Fifteen-second pause minimum
I want you to concentrate on your breathing again
Pause
Notice as you breathe
Pause
On each out-breath you feel more and more relaxed
Long pause
I would like you in your mind to say a number of your choice such as the number one
Pause (if the number evokes an emotion in you choose another number)
And say it every time you breathe out
Long pause
This will help you to push away any unwanted thoughts you may have
Pause
Each time you breathe out just say the number in your mind

Thirty-second pause
I want you now
Pause
To think of your favourite relaxing place
Long pause
Try and see it in your mind's eye
Long pause
Look at the colours
Long pause
Now focus on one colour
Long pause
Now concentrate on any sounds or noises in your favourite relaxing place. If there are no sounds, then focus on the silence
Long pause
Now concentrate on any smells or aromas in your favourite relaxing place
Long pause
Now just imagine touching something
Pause
In your favourite relaxing place
Long pause
Just imagine how it feels
Long pause
I want you now to concentrate on your breathing again
Pause
Notice once again that every time you breathe out
Pause
You feel more
Pause
And more relaxed
Long pause
Whenever you want to in the future you will be able to remember your favourite place or the breathing exercise and it will help you to relax quickly
Long pause
In a few moments' time, but not quite yet, I'm going to count to three
Pause
And you will be able to open your eyes in your own time
Pause (or insert, 'go off to sleep', if you so wish)
One
Pause
Two
Pause
Three
Pause

Open your eyes in your own time

In our experience, we have found this multimodal method of relaxation to be particularly useful for people suffering from anxiety, tension headaches, high blood pressure, insomnia, and Type A behaviour; and it can help control general irritability experienced by someone on a 'stop smoking' programme. However, care should be taken if you suffer from asthma, epilepsy or panic attacks because relaxation can exacerbate these conditions in rare cases.

If you are interested in finding out more about relaxation, yoga or meditation, you might like to contact your local adult education service which may run classes. Alternatively, a local sports centre may run classes.

© Stephen Palmer, 1993

RETIREMENT

Although you may be considering setting up in private practice in the immediate future, the long-term future is also worth considering at this stage. Whether it is your pension, putting aside savings, moving on retirement to another location, or downsizing, it is worth spending a while just thinking about what your hopes and goals are for your retirement, as this may influence what you do now, or at some time over the next decade or so, depending upon your age. Certainly the UK government has warned us that many of us are not saving enough for our retirement. You may wish to continue working part-time as a counsellor, psychotherapist or psychologist in retirement to support your lifestyle and/or keep you stimulated, but this may depend upon your health.

CONCLUSION

In this final part of the book, we have provided you with a wide range of different techniques and strategies to help you consider a number of personal issues relating to setting up a practice: cognitive thinking skills, imagery, managing stress, time management, and relaxation. Setting up in private practice may be straightforward. However, our approach is to be prepared and in this part of the book we have shared with you the overall approach that we have found to help us to deal successfully with real and imagined problems.

Postscript

You may now have finished reading this book. Some of you may believe that you are now well prepared to start on the new, exciting and challenging journey of private practice. However, some of you may still feel concerned that it could be too much of a challenge to tackle. This is understandable. You may wish to spend more time in the planning phase and receive some professional guidance too.

We have attempted to cover the main issues involved with private practice, including the personal aspects that can create additional stress for us if we are not prepared to meet the internal and external challenges. This book has used the self-coaching model whereby we encourage the reader to plan, prepare and then act. The action can be taken alone or with the support of colleagues, professionals, family and friends. Breaking down the tasks involved in setting up in private practice into small manageable steps makes the overall goals easier.

We do not believe that we need to wish you good luck on your journey, as we have found that hard work and practice seem to bring their own good luck. Do let us know how you have progressed in setting up and running your private practice.

References

Barrow, P., 2001, *The Best-Laid Business Plans: How to Write Them, How to Pitch Them*, London, Virgin Business Guides.

Benson, H., 1976, *The Relaxation Response*, London, Collins.

Berne, E., 1966, *Principles of Group Treatment*, New York, Grove Press.

Bond, T., 2000, *Standards and Ethics for Counselling in Action*, London, Sage.

Bongar, B. *et al* (eds), 1998, *Risk Management with Suicidal Patients*, New York, Guilford Press.

Bor, R. and Watts, M. (eds), 1999, *The Trainee Handbook*, London, Sage.

Caird, S., 1993, 'What Do Psychological Tests Suggest About Entrepreneurs?', *Journal of Managerial Psychology*, 8, 6.

Clark, J. (ed.), 2002, *Freelance Counselling and Psychotherapy*, Hove, Brunner-Routledge.

Cooper, C. and Palmer, S., 2001, *Conquer Your Stress*, London, CIPD.

Covey, S., 1989, *The Seven Habits of Highly Effective People*, London, Simon & Schuster.

Daines, B., Gask, L. and Usherwood, T., 1997, *Medical and Psychiatric Issues for Therapists*, London, Sage.

Dryden, W. and Feltham, C., 1994, *Developing the Practice of Counselling*, London, Sage.

Falloon, V., 1992, *How to Get More Clients*, London, Brainwave Publications.

Gordon, L., 1984, *Survey of Personal Values (Examiner's Manual)*, Iowa, Science Research Associates.

Guy, J.D., 1987, *The Personal Life of the Psychotherapist*, New York, Wiley.

Harold, S.A., 2002, *Marketing for Complementary Therapists*, Plymouth, How To Books.

Howard, S., 1999, *Creating a Successful CV*, London, Dorling Kindersley.

Jenkins, P., 1997, *Counselling, Psychotherapy and the Law*, London, Sage.

Jenkins, P., 2002, *Legal Issues in Counselling and Psychotherapy*, London, Sage.

Johns, H. (ed.), 1998, *Balancing Acts: Studies in Counselling Training*, London, Routledge.

Jung, C., 1966, 'The Psychology of Transference', in *The Practice of Psychotherapy*, Vol. 16, Princeton, Princeton University Press.

Keenan, D., 1995, *English Law*, London, Pitman.

McMahon, G., 1994, *Setting Up Your Own Private Practice in Counselling and Psychotherapy*, Cambridge, NEC.

McMullin, R.E., 1986, *Handbook of Cognitive Techniques*, New York, Norton.

Milner, P. and Palmer, S. (eds), 2001, *The BACP Counselling Reader*, London, Sage.

Palmer, S., 1993, *Multimodal Techniques: Relaxation and Hypnosis*, London, Centre for Stress Management and Centre for Multimodal Therapy.

Palmer, S., 2002, 'Confidentiality: A Case Study', in P. Jenkins (ed.) *Legal Issues in Counselling and Psychotherapy*, London, Sage.

Palmer, S. and Dryden, W., 1995, *Counselling for Stress Problems*, London, Sage.

Palmer, S. and McMahon, G., 1997, *Client Assessment*, London, Sage.

Palmer, S. and Neenan, M., 1998, 'Double Imagery Procedure', *The Rational Emotive Behaviour Therapist*, 6, 2: 89–92.

Palmer, S. and Strickland, L., 1996, *Stress Management: A Quick Guide*, Dunstable, Folens.

Palmer, S. and Szymanska, K., 1994, 'Cognitive Therapy and Counselling', in *The BACP Counselling Reader*, London, Sage.

Palmer, S. and Whybrow, A., 2004, *Coaching Training Manual*, London, Centre for Coaching.

Palmer, S., Cooper, C. and Thomas, K., 2003, *Creating a Balance: Managing Stress*, London, British Library.

Sills, C. (ed.), 1997, *Contracts in Counselling*, London, Sage.

Syme, G., 1994, *Counselling in Independent Practice*, Buckingham, Open University Press.

Truman, M., 1997, *Teach Yourself Book-Keeping and Accounting for Your Small Business*, Teach Yourself Series, London, British Institute of Management.

Ward, E., King, M., Lloyd, M., Bower, P. Sibbald, B., Farrelly, S., Gabbay, M., Tarrier, N. and Addington-Hall, J., 2000, 'Randomised controlled trial of non-directive counselling, cognitive-behaviour therapy and usual general practitioner care for patients with depression. I Clinical Effectiveness'. *British Medical Journal* 321: 1383–1388.

Whiteley, J., 2002, *Small Business Tax Guide*, London, How To Reference.

Wilkins, P., 1997, *Personal and Professional Development for Therapists*, London, Sage.

Recommended reading

LEGAL AND ETHICAL ISSUES

Legal Issues in Counselling and Psychotherapy, Peter Jenkins, 2002, Sage Publications, London.
Law for the Small Business, Patricia Clayton, 2001, Business Enterprise Guides, Kogan Page, London.
Counselling, Psychotherapy and the Law, Peter Jenkins, 1997, Sage Publications, London.
Standards and Ethics for Counselling in Action, Tim Bond, 2000, Sage Publications, London.
Ethical Framework for Good Practice in Counselling and Psychotherapy, British Association for Counselling and Psychotherapy, 1 Regent Place, Rugby, Warwickshire CV21 2PJ, 0870 443 5252, www.bacp.co.uk

SUPERVISION

Counselling Supervision: Theory, Skills and Practice, Michael Carroll, 1996, Cassell, London.
Making the Most of Supervision, Francesca Inskipp and Brigid Procter, 1994, Cascade Publications, Twickenham.

PROFESSIONAL ISSUES

Personal and Professional Development for Counsellors, Paul Wilkins, 1997, Sage Publications, London.
Client Assessment, Stephen Palmer and Gladeana McMahon, 1997, Sage Publications, London.
Risk Management with Suicidal Patients, Bruce Bongar, Alan Berman, Ronald Maris, Morton Silverman, Eric Harris and Wendy Packman, 1998, Guilford Press, New York.
Medical and Psychiatric Issues for Counsellors, Brian Daines, Linda Gask and Tim Usherwood, 1997, Sage Publications, London.
Contracts in Counselling, Charlotte Sills, 1997, Sage Publications, London.
Suicide: Strategies and Interventions for Reduction and Prevention, Stephen Palmer, 2006, Routledge, London.

PRIVATE PRACTICE

Freelance Counselling and Psychotherapy, Jean Clark, 2002, Brunner-Routledge, London.

BUSINESS ISSUES

Marketing for Complementary Therapists, Steven A. Harold, 2002, How To Books, Oxford.

PERSONAL DEVELOPMENT

Conquer Your Stress, Cary Cooper and Stephen Palmer, 2000, CIPD, London.
Creating a Balance: Managing Stress, Stephen Palmer, Cary Cooper and Kate Thomas, 2003, British
    Library, London.

Useful addresses

OFFICIAL ORGANISATIONS

Data Protection Registrar
Wycliffe House
Water Lane
Wilmslow
Cheshire
SK9 5AF
01625 545 745 (enquiries)
01625 535 711 (admin.)
www.dataprotection.gov.uk

Customs and Excise
London Central Office
Berkeley House
304 Regents Park Road
Finchley
London
N3 2JY
020 7865 4400
www.hmce.gov.uk

Inland Revenue
www.inlandrevenue.gov.uk

INSURANCE COMPANY

Towergate SMG Professional Risks
31 Clarendon Road
Leeds
LS2 9PA
0113 294 4000

THERAPISTS' ORGANISATIONS

British Association for Counselling and Psychotherapy (BACP)
1 Regent Place
Rugby
Warwickshire
CV21 2PJ
0870 443 5252
www.bacp.co.uk

British Psychological Society (BPS)
St Andrew's House
48 Princess Road East
Leicester
LE1 7DR
01162 549 568
www.bps.org.uk

United Kingdom Council for Psychotherapy (UKCP)
167–169 Great Portland Street
London
N1 5SB
020 7436 3002

Confederation of Scottish Counselling Agencies (COSCA)
18 Viewfield Street
Stirling
FK8 1UA

Irish Association for Counselling and Therapy (IACT)
8 Cumberland Street
Dun Laoghaire
Co. Dublin
Ireland

European Association of Counselling
PO Box 6699
Dublin 2
Ireland

TRAINING IN SETTING UP IN PRIVATE PRACTICE

Centre for Stress Management
156 Westcombe Hill
London
SE3 7DH
020 8293 4334
www.managingstress.com

ACCOUNTANTS

Association of Chartered Certified Accountants (ACCA)
64 Finnieston Square
Glasgow
United Kingdom
G3 8DT
General Enquiries: info@accaglobal.com
Student Enquiries: students@accaglobal.com
Member Enquiries: members@accaglobal.com
Website: http://www.acca.co.uk
tel: +44 (0)141 582 2000
fax: +44 (0)141 582 2222

Institite of Chartered Accountants
Chartered Acountants' Hall
PO Box 433
London
EC2P 2BJ
020 7920 8100
www.icaew.co.uk

Index

Client Information Sheet 72, 74; collection of 39; guilt over 2; legal issues 69–70; marketing aspects 55; provision for savings 63; socio-economic status of clients 15; *see also* income
finance 33–6; business plan 22–9; financial control 7; pensions 15, 26, 28, 43, 61–4, 65; record-keeping 13, 37–9, 41–3, 45; *see also* expenditure; income; tax issues
flexible thinking 116
follow-up 51–2
fortune-telling 108, 113, 123
friends 12, 65
frustration tolerance 116
furniture 57, 58–9
further education 14

general practitioners (GPs) 16, 47, 94, 98–9, 101
generalisation 116
gifts 77
government-funded initiatives 14
GPs *see* general practitioners
grants 14
guaranteed sessional work 30, 31–2

Harvey-Jones, John 10
headaches 134
health centres 107, 108
HFT *see* high frustration tolerance
high blood pressure 134
high frustration tolerance (HFT) 116
Hinch, Kate 127
holidays 23, 26, 36, 51
home working 56–7, 58, 105; financial issues 26, 27, 41; insurance issues 59; stress issues 107, 108; *see also* premises
hours of work 31, 49, 109, 126; *see also* time management
Howard, Simon 19

'I can't stand it' error 116
illness 36, 60, 105, 107
image 50, 52–4
imagery: coping 125–6; motivation 126; relaxation 130
income 6–7, 31, 33–6; accountants 13; bank statements 40; business plan 15, 22–9; business/personal separation 37;

drawings 43; irregularity of 107; record-keeping 37; tax liability 43–4; *see also* fees
indemnity insurance 60, 68
Inland Revenue 13–14, 40, 41; *see also* tax issues
insomnia 134
insurance 43, 59–60, 78
Internet 16, 19, 42
invoicing 39, 45, 70
irritability 134
ISAs 61, 62, 63

journals 42, 69, 90

Keenan, D. 71
knowledge 11, 17, 88

labelling 110, 111
lecturing 97
legal issues 67–82; confidentiality 68–9; contracts 71–4; court cases 68, 78–80; fees 69–70; partnerships 32; renting premises 58; Small Claims Court 45, 70, 77–8; storage of records 80–2; suicidal clients 101
letters 93–4
LFT *see* low frustration tolerance
local authorities 14
location 9, 19, 20–1, 46, 99; *see also* environment; premises
logical thinking 10
low frustration tolerance (LFT) 116

McMahon, Gladeana 1, 47–8
magnification 112
Making Choices Form 104, 105–6
malpractice 32, 50, 60
market forces 11
market research 46–9
marketing 46–56; *see also* advertising; publicity
medical back-up 98–9
mental illness 98
mind-reading 112, 119
minimisation 112
mission statement 18
motivation 8, 10, 107, 110, 118, 126
motor costs 42
Multimodal Relaxation Method 130–4

national campaigns 54